NO SEX

Spiritual Path Self-Publishing
Black Experience Magazine, LLC

NO SEX

ISBN: 978-1-387-64659-3

Published by arrangement with Black Experience Magazine, LLC

Portions of this book first appeared in Black Experience Magazine, © Spiritual Path Self-Publishing Company, 2010

First Printing: October, 2022

TABLE OF CONTENTS

I encourage you to really pay attention to your own needs and either change how you feel about the lack of sexual frequency or change the relationship.

You are the only one responsible for yourself and you deserve a satisfying sexual relationship.

PREFACE

Why sex matters so much in a relationship – and can cause so many problems. From a certain age onwards, sex is a major part of most people's lives. It can give us so much joy – but also seems to cause so much trouble.

Why is that? Why can sex seem to have so much power over us and be so important?

Perhaps to understand the answer to this, the first thing is to consider why we want to have sex and what benefits it gives us.

These are emotional, spiritual, and physical in their nature. There are undoubtedly physical reasons why people want to have sex. After all, it is how we are designed: to ensure the human race continues.

So, sex gives us pleasurable physical feelings. Nothing else gives us these same sorts of physical feelings. They are inundating and there to encourage us to want to have sex.

There is also an emotional and spiritual drive for and reasons to have sex. One thing is that it releases our happiness hormones, and this increases our bond with someone. Sex boosts intimacy between people because it is as intimate as it gets. To be naked as we mostly are during sex is a vulnerable act of trust in another person.

Sex is a very spiritual act too. It is two people becoming one with each other. It is a way of showing love and affection for another person. It is literally a part of "making love" – as in creating and making love grow.

It boosts security in a relationship. It shows a strong commitment to each other. A healthy sex life shows that partners are in tune with each other. It is that their communication is good and or that compromise, as is needed in many ways in all relationships, is positive.

It is also a great way of relieving stress. This is to do with hormones that are released during sex and particularly at climax. But it is also because it is something that stops us from thinking and worrying about anything else.

We are, naturally, in the moment. It is an escape.

For this reason, sex is sometimes called "la petite mort" in France – meaning "the little death". This is because we lose ourselves so much during sex it is as though the ego has died. Again, this is why sex is a very spiritual thing.

We are all on a journey toward better. If you've struggled with sexual temptation, maybe you've wondered why sexual desire is so difficult to resist, or even wondered why did God create sex?

You're not alone in wondering. Parents wring their hands as they watch their kids walk into a world pushing sex at them, husbands and wives wonder if their beloved will be faithful, and people the world over are sounding alarms over the very real problems of rape, sexual abuse, and sex trafficking.

Wouldn't it have been better if God had designed sex with a little less power, created sexual desire with just a bit less voltage?

I've felt the iron grip of lust refuse to let me go when I was trying to break free from sexual addiction. I've got kids and know that helpless feeling of watching them walk into a school prescribing condoms and affirming sexual confusion. And some of my earliest memories are of family members weeping over infidelity.

Sexual and romantic desires have the power to break hearts, enslave bodies, and wreck the world.

So why on earth did God create sex so powerful? I want to unpack this a bit because it will help all of us to better navigate this sex saturated culture.

Sex was powerful before sin entered the picture. In fact, sex was more powerful then. The atomic power of sex is not something the evil one invented, not something he would ever even dream of, Sex is God's invention and he loves what he has made.

What we object to most is not the power of sex, but the power of sin. Whether how we eat, drink, marry, parent, work, or play, sin hijacks the power of good and steers it destructively.

Sex is one of the most important areas of humanity Jesus came to "seek and to save" (Luke 19:10). He didn't come to extinguish sexual desire. He didn't come to pull the plug and shut the whole thing down. Sin has done that! Jesus came to plug it back in, to restore all the love and life and joy and glory and power that sex is meant to have.

So, in whatever way, sex feels too powerful in your life, begin by bringing all your sexual addictions, fears, hurts, and sorrows—sins you've done and sins done to you—to Jesus. And keep bringing them. He has come not to condemn but to save. Trust him to do so.

365 DAYS, NO SEX

God made sex to give us vision beyond the physical pleasure of sex. There is so much more to sexual intimacy between husband and wife. When the Holy Spirit resides in you, all of life has a spiritual essence which includes sexual intimacy.

"Where there is no revelation [no vision -KJV], people cast off restraint [perish – KJV]; but blessed is the one who heeds wisdom's instruction," Proverbs 29:19 (NIV).

He Asked 365 Times but She Said No Sex!

I need some advice in regards to my sex life. I have been in a relationship with this amazing wife for about 10 years but the last 365 days I have not been able get me sum. I really care about her with all my heart and feel she feel the same. But then, whenever I feel like having sex with her, she just says no. The last time we had sex was 365 day ago.

I have tried my best and have tried everything to make her have sex with me. For example, I kiss her passionately, I buy her gifts, take her out for dinners, walks, give her surprises but that's it. She feels very happy with these things but doesn't feel like having sex. I feel so frustrated all the time because of lack of intimacy and sex.

I have also tried touching her but she doesn't allow me to touch anything of hers except for boobs but sometime I can't do that too. I try to arouse her by trying to give her an orgasm but she always has reasons such as she isn't shaved or hasn't taken a shower or doesn't smell good or she feels tickled and so I should refrain from touching her vagina.

365 DAYS, NO SEX

God made sex to give us vision beyond the physical pleasure of sex. There is so much more to sexual intimacy between husband and wife. When the Holy Spirit resides in you, all of life has a spiritual essence which includes sexual intimacy.

"Where there is no revelation [no vision -KJV], people cast off restraint [perish – KJV]; but blessed is the one who heeds wisdom's instruction," Proverbs 29:19 (NIV).

He Asked 365 Times but She Said No Sex!

I need some advice in regards to my sex life. I have been in a relationship with this amazing wife for about 10 years but the last 365 days I have not been able get me sum. I really care about her with all my heart and feel she feel the same. But then, whenever I feel like having sex with her, she just says no. The last time we had sex was 365 day ago.

I have tried my best and have tried everything to make her have sex with me. For example, I kiss her passionately, I buy her gifts, take her out for dinners, walks, give her surprises but that's it. She feels very happy with these things but doesn't feel like having sex. I feel so frustrated all the time because of lack of intimacy and sex.

I have also tried touching her but she doesn't allow me to touch anything of hers except for boobs but sometime I can't do that too. I try to arouse her by trying to give her an orgasm but she always has reasons such as she isn't shaved or hasn't taken a shower or doesn't smell good or she feels tickled and so I should refrain from touching her vagina.

PREFACE

Why sex matters so much in a relationship – and can cause so many problems. From a certain age onwards, sex is a major part of most people's lives. It can give us so much joy – but also seems to cause so much trouble.

Why is that? Why can sex seem to have so much power over us and be so important?

Perhaps to understand the answer to this, the first thing is to consider why we want to have sex and what benefits it gives us.

These are emotional, spiritual, and physical in their nature. There are undoubtedly physical reasons why people want to have sex. After all, it is how we are designed: to ensure the human race continues.

So, sex gives us pleasurable physical feelings. Nothing else gives us these same sorts of physical feelings. They are inundating and there to encourage us to want to have sex.

There is also an emotional and spiritual drive for and reasons to have sex. One thing is that it releases our happiness hormones, and this increases our bond with someone. Sex boosts intimacy between people because it is as intimate as it gets. To be naked as we mostly are during sex is a vulnerable act of trust in another person.

Sex is a very spiritual act too. It is two people becoming one with each other. It is a way of showing love and affection for another person. It is literally a part of "making love" – as in creating and making love grow.

It boosts security in a relationship. It shows a strong commitment to each other. A healthy sex life shows that partners are in tune with each other. It is that their communication is good and or that compromise, as is needed in many ways in all relationships, is positive.

It is also a great way of relieving stress. This is to do with hormones that are released during sex and particularly at climax. But it is also because it is something that stops us from thinking and worrying about anything else.

We are, naturally, in the moment. It is an escape.

For this reason, sex is sometimes called "la petite mort" in France – meaning "the little death". This is because we lose ourselves so much during sex it is as though the ego has died. Again, this is why sex is a very spiritual thing.

We are all on a journey toward better. If you've struggled with sexual temptation, maybe you've wondered why sexual desire is so difficult to resist, or even wondered why did God create sex?

You're not alone in wondering. Parents wring their hands as they watch their kids walk into a world pushing sex at them, husbands and wives wonder if their beloved will be faithful, and people the world over are sounding alarms over the very real problems of rape, sexual abuse, and sex trafficking.

Wouldn't it have been better if God had designed sex with a little less power, created sexual desire with just a bit less voltage?

I've felt the iron grip of lust refuse to let me go when I was trying to break free from sexual addiction. I've got kids and

know that helpless feeling of watching them w
prescribing condoms and affirming sexual
some of my earliest memories are of family m
over infidelity.

Sexual and romantic desires have the power
enslave bodies, and wreck the world.

So why on earth did God create sex so pow
unpack this a bit because it will help all of us t
this sex saturated culture.

Sex was powerful before sin entered the picture.
more powerful then. The atomic power of sex i
the evil one invented, not something he would
of, Sex is God's invention and he loves what h

What we object to most is not the power of se
of sin. Whether how we eat, drink, marry, paren
sin hijacks the power of good and steers it dest

Sex is one of the most important areas of huma
to "seek and to save" (Luke 19:10). He
extinguish sexual desire. He didn't come to p
shut the whole thing down. Sin has done that!
plug it back in, to restore all the love and life an
and power that sex is meant to have.

So, in whatever way, sex feels too powerful in
by bringing all your sexual addictions, fea
sorrows—sins you've done and sins done to
And keep bringing them. He has come not to
save. Trust him to do so.

I feel so rejected and frustrated because I always tell her that I don't care whether she is shaved or not or whether she has taken a shower or not. She is always super clean though and smells really good all the time, so I guess it is just in her head and that makes her say no. Moreover, she never touches me. She feels super shy and weird to touch my dick any more to arouse me, let alone giving me a head that just stop altogether. I have never demanded a blowjob but I expect her to play along and do something.

I have already talked to her like 20 plus times about how I feel and the last time I talked to her, I told her that I feel like breaking up with her because I feel frustrated. I am always watching porn and satisfying myself while she sleeps next to me. So much that I have stopped making efforts for sex because I know she will say no again.

I know she isn't seeing anyone else and is not cheating because she is deeply in love with me and wants to be with me forever but then, I cannot see myself without sex for the rest of my life.

The stage has reached where we take showers together to reignite our sex life but I feel nothing. In fact, I feel like I would be giving in to a pity sex.

Please advise what should I do? I love her a lot and don't feel like leaving her because she is super sweet and all but then I don't know if I can continue with just sweetness. I need some action as well."

I decided to not break-up with my wife and give her another chance. However, 365 days down the line the situation is the same. Though these 365 days haven't been easy and we have had a few fights and took some time off each other as well. But we always came back and talked and it was during one of these talks that something very weird came up.

I asked my wife whether she feels like having sex at all or not. I was direct and asked her if she was masturbating or not. She told me that she was not masturbating on an average three times per week when I was at work or playing with the kids. I don't get it. If she is feeling horny, why not be with me and have sex? Rather, she preferred doing it alone.

Now, I am getting frustrated with all this. I am thinking of ending this completely. Please advise whether there is anything else that I can do to save this. Her masturbation thing has really got me thinking and worried of my future.

When you're in a relationship, sometimes one side of the couple just doesn't feel like having sex. How many times has your girlfriend turned down your advances because 1) she has her period, 2) she's not in the mood, or 3) she hates you? It happens.

I kept track of all the reasons my wife said no to Sex for 365 days. Here are some reasons she said "It's too hot" 15 times, followed by "It's too cold" three times, "Pretending to sleep" 35 times, "I'm too drunk" 17 times and the weirdest one..."It will make the cat jealous" 18 times???? WTF is that even a thing?

They also say "I'm not in the mood today", "I don't feel like doing it now", "I got a splitting headache", "I am on my periods," etc, etc, etc. It's unfortunate that even today women need to make up stories to say no to having sex. Why is a blatant and direct 'no' not enough? If women say no, men feel agitated. To put it straight, they take it on their masculinity, because who cares about consent anyway, right? Some men feel hurt which leads to women trying to deal with it tactfully with excuses that look as genuine as possible.

1. I've got a headache/feel sick. Ah, the most common excuse of all time. Ah, the most common excuse of all time. It's perfectly understandable if she actually has a headache, because sex isn't much fun if she has pounding head while you're pounding away. But if she's been using the same excuse every day for the past 2 weeks, she either really needs to see a doctor, or she flat out doesn't want to have sex with you. That's up to you to figure out.

2. I'm too busy. Apparently, 75% of couples blame their crazy work schedules and hectic lives on their lack of interest in sex. If she doesn't have time for herself, she's probably not going to have time to have sex with you, either. In this scenario, try as a couple to set aside time for getting intimate with each other. Instead of bumming out watching Netflix together, upgrade that to Netflix and chill. Problem solved.

3. I'm too tired. When she's tired, she's not going to feel like getting busy. So, take a nap together, or treat her to a double espresso with a lot of sugar, because then she won't be too tired to have sex with you. It's a win-win situation.

4. I don't have an orgasm so what's the point? This is all on you, my friend. If she's getting nothing out of sex, she'd much rather keep her panties on and not have a sweaty man flopping around on top of her. You can't really blame her for that. In this case, it's best to try different things in the bedroom to make sure she orgasms too, like going down on her more, experimenting a little, or just having sex outside of the bedroom in some exotic locale, like the kitchen. It's more exciting.

5. I feel fat. Sorry to say, but this is a legit reason for a woman to not want to get naked, because when a woman feels fat,

she sure as hell doesn't feel sexy. And when she doesn't feel sexy, she won't want to take her clothes off. You know what I mean?

If your lady sobs that she's fat when you try to get things hot and heavy, just tell her she's the most beautiful woman you've ever seen. And actually, mean it. It might work. Or, just have a lighter dinner from then on, and she won't feel like a whale afterwards.

6. I'm sick of being hassled for sex If you're the one constantly initiating sex, she's going to get bored, which might be why she's giving you this excuse. If you're the one constantly initiating sex, she's going to get bored, which might be why she's giving you this excuse.

    "It's called 'the see-saw phenomenon': the more one person does, the less the other does. The more often they initiate sex, the less often you will," implying that the more you ask her for sex, the less interested she's going to be. "Here's what you do to fix this one: tell your partner you miss not being the one to initiate sex. This alone – and I guarantee it – will have an extraordinary reaction," See, easy fix!

7. I'm bored stupid She needs some excitement! Buy some sex toys, try different positions, surprise her with a trip south of the border *wink wink* and she'll reciprocate like crazy. Trust us. Getting passion and excitement back into your sex life isn't that difficult – just introduce some novel things to the bedroom, and voila. Problem solved.

8. I simply can't be bothered Yikes, this is bad. She's over you and your penis. Either she's cheating on you, or she doesn't miss having sex with you, "The less sex you have,

the less you miss it," which raises the question, how often are you having sex with her?

As a solution, "Consider scheduling sex sessions – it doesn't work for all couples but it works for more than you think." And if that doesn't work, the relationship may well be over. Sorry.

9. "I am on my periods." - Let's admit it ladies, we all have used this one and no other excuse works better to keep sex at bay. No matter how much we hate to use menstruation as an excuse to not have sex, but we do.

10. You Have a Visit from "Aunt Flow" - The excuse to shut down all excuses — telling your date that you're on your period is a sure-fire way to get out of a date. If he knows this, then he knows his chances of getting some are nil.

   This could be a great way to see if sex is all he was after in the first place. Kudos to you for dodging a bullet with this excuse!

11. "God, I overate, I feel bloated!" - Of course, you are feeling uneasy and your tummy hurts at the thought of any action. But what's even more uneasy is to not be able to say NO to sex directly because we have to be considerate about your feelings.

12. "I am married!" - Well, in a bar when women often stumble upon men lurking around trying to fulfil their sexual needs, women put an end to the conversation with just one statement--"I am married." Even better if they say, "I have kids." What world are we living in? Argh!

13. "I have a urinary tract infection." - Because you can't really question a UT

14. "I got a severe back pain." - Perks of using your back pain as an excuse is you get a back massage instead and a lot of pampering. Now who doesn't want that? A good massage is any day better than faking an orgasm, right?

15. Am still breastfeeding: Breastfeeding should not be allowed to affect your sex life with your husband. Medically sex can take place within three and six months after birth. What is required is to allow time for the cervix to close, postpartum bleeding to stop, and any tears or repaired lacerations to heal.

16. The other important timeline is your own. Some women feel ready to resume sex within a few weeks of giving birth, while others need a few months. Some women do say the child will be sucking the father's spermatozoa but that is not true because it has no direct relationship with breastfeeding

17. Am praying: Some wives are too spiritual when it comes to sex, they will always pretend to be praying whenever they notice advancement from their husband.

18. Not in the mood: You don't have to be in the mood before you can allow your husband to sleep with you. Sex is one of the obligations to your husband for the sustainability of your marriage. It is a ministry of purification to make your husband pure.

19. I am not happy: Some wives will only permit sex with their husband when they are happy. If you only allow that to be daily occurrence in your marriage it will definitely ruin it.

20. Bring up issues: Time for sex is not the appropriate time to start bringing up issues like the school fees yet unpaid, the house rent and other inappropriate discussions. All these will affect the moral of the man

21. I came home late: If you have the kind of job that normally causes you to come home late you need to look how to go around it. Your husband may be enduring it but it will never good for the health of your marriage

22. I just took communion: Taking communion in the church should not be allowed to deprive you of sleeping with your husband, what you want to do is not sinful it is God that instituted marriage and purposely put sex in the middle of the marriage

23. Just to punish your husband; Sex should never be used as a weapon but for pleasure within the marriage

24. It Is Raining: Some wives said when they sleep with their husband during the raining season the unborn baby may have pneumonia. Tell me when it is the best time to have it than when it is raining.

25. The sun is shining there will be heat. some concluded if you have sex with your husband and eventually become pregnant you may give birth to an albino.

26. I am only the one doing the house chores: although house chores and kitchen work is not labeled for women only. But if your husband fails to support you either in the kitchen or doing the house chores that doesn't mean you should retaliate by depriving him of sleeping with you. Doing this

will aggravate the issues instead of that you look for appropriate time and discuss it.

27. "I'm angry with you" - Some sneaky devils try and avoid sex by dragging out an argument for longer than it needed to last or purposely causing one.

    We've all heard of the scenario; you're having a fantastic evening watching films, gorging on a candle-lit romantic meal, and laughing at each other's jokes when suddenly the bedroom part comes and boom - you just remembered your argument from the other night.

    Suddenly the candles are blown out, the oversized comfy pajamas have made their grand entrance and you're lying on the bed facing opposite directions. No sex tonight.

28. I just had my hair done.

29. She just picks a fight before bedtime.

30. Why don't we just cuddle. That's much more romantic.

31. It's not your birthday!

32. You want sex and I want the dog walked. Do that with any regularity and then we can talk.

33. Have you been drinking? I can smell the alcohol coming out of your pores and it is making me nauseated.

34. I'm think I have bronchitis or strep or something. If I gave you a blow job, I might infect your penis.

35. I have to get up early in the morning.

36. I'm having a Pap Smear tomorrow and want it unsoiled.

37. But it's not Saturday or Wednesday?

38. "We should have come to bed half an hour earlier if you wanted to do this tonight."

39. I pulled a muscle in my leg, the pain is killing me. This can actually give you a few days off.

40. I am too tired. Tomorrow, hopefully I should be ok.

It's easy to find excuses not to have sex. The problem lies in finding one that your partner will actually believe and can't be disproven easily.

Remember to consider each excuse carefully before using it, and when possible, be honest! Honesty is essential in any relationship. If you find yourself making excuses, then you might need to have a talk with your partner.

SEX FOR 365 DAYS STRAIGHT

Relationship with my husband and my body is incredibly changed. Now, three years later, we still have sex every night, says Ayana. Ayana Wilkinson, a mother of three from Ayana, honestly told why she decided to have sex every day for a year.

She reveals that she did it, and only for herself, because one day, when she looks in the mirror, something inside her snapped. "Three years ago, I had sex every day and it lasted a year. I immediately preempt your questions no, it was not with 365 different men, but only one my husband. And yes, even when I had my period. I have no idea what my kids are doing while I'm having sex. And finally, no, I did not do that to save my marriage, but to preserve myself".

Shortly after I gave birth for the third time, I remember that I went out of the tub, I saw myself in the mirror and asked myself: 'What is my mother doing in the bathroom?' 'From that moment on, I did not allow myself to be naked. I extinguished the lights during sex, clothing skirt stomach and chest and was waiting for my husband to leave the room to changed dress.

As the years passed, the absence of my naked body began to worry me. Is my husband Julies still remembered what I look like naked? It crossed my mind to have sex every night, year after discussions with a friend who is also doing it every night.

The idea of having sex every day a year sounded repulsive to me, but also somewhat intriguing because it made me look at my naked body every day. The sheets will surely at some point move and the lights will stay on, right?

Julies is, as I expected, immediately agreed and the whole year, except for when we were traveling, a stomach virus separated, we had sex. The beginning was difficult. The thought that every night I need to have sex before going to sleep, and that I worked all day and struggled with four children, I was very strained. I wanted to be just hatched on the bed, eating cereal and watching TV.

But as the months passed, I began to look forward to it. Sex has become more than sex and some special feelings are awakened.

We were more romantic, we touched and kissed more passionately every morning before going to work. Our relationship has become stronger and better because under the sheets all flourished.

Again, I enjoyed the sex and in my body and I finally stopped hiding my physical shortcomings and eagerly accepted them. For the first time, I was burdened with the fact that sex is better, but whether my stomach from this angle, it looks smaller.

After a year, I stopped completely to wear clothes. Relaxed I walked naked to the bathroom, preparing lunch in their underwear. The connection with my husband and my body changed to an amazing way.

Now, three years later, we still have sex every night. Oh dear, I'm kidding, of course not! From all this we learned how much sex we need in order to be happy in marriage and that there is no end of the world if you pass two weeks without sex. I have learned that I am a better wife, a better mother and a better woman when I was sure of myself and I feel good about myself.

Regular sex in marriage does not seem resistant to divorce or immune to infidelity, but it helps me to get more confidence. In the end, it was never about someone wants me, but I want myself. And it took me only a year of sex to see that.

WHAT IS A SEXLESS RELATIONSHIP?

A sexless relationship is a relationship in which there is little to no sexual activity between the partners. Many couples experience periods of more sex and less sex. A temporary period of less sex isn't typically considered "sexless." While there is no official definition, many define a sexless relationship as one in which the couple has not had sex (or has had only extremely infrequent sex) for a year or more.

There are many possible reasons a couple might find themselves in a sexless partnership. Whether being in a sexless relationship is an issue depends on the couple, but if the lack of sex and physical intimacy is a problem, there are ways to work through it together and separately starting with identifying the underlying cause.

Is having sex once per month considered a sexless relationship?

A sexless relationship is one in which sex has not happened for 1 year or greater. A low-sex relationship is one that is having sex 10 times a year or less. So, a relationship that is having sex roughly once a month does not meet either of these definitions.

However, that may provide you little comfort if you believe having sex once a month is not enough. Having sex one time a month is not inherently a problem. That level of sexual frequency is only problematic if the couple sees it as problematic.

If a couple is only having sex one time per month, it may not provide the couple enough time together to be able to experience a full sexually intimate connection.

HOW OFTEN SHOULD COUPLES HAVE SEX?

This is hard to say because each couple is so different. Some couples do best when they have sex daily. Other couples prefer weekly or every other week. There are even couples that prefer to not have sex at all.

Resident sex therapist Dr. Kyle Zrenchik recommends couples to have sex no less than 1-2 times every 1-2 weeks to ensure that they are experiencing enough sexual intimacy.

Sexual intimacy, as Dr. Zrenchik states, is more than just sexual frequency. "It involves sharing emotions, being vulnerable, and taking risks. Also, it involves experiencing something inside the bedroom that is different and special.

Sexual intimacy provides a vehicle for connection and relationship building that cannot be replicated in any other way.

Both emotional and sexual intimacy are crucial factors that affect a couple's overall relationship quality.

Ultimately, it is up to the couple to determine their ideal sexual frequency. As long as the couple feels sexually connected and satisfied, then the number is largely irrelevant.

"Somehow my husband's interest in sex decreased dramatically immediately after relationship."

"So, in the early years of my relationship, we had a lot of issues with [not having sex]. Somehow my husband's interest in sex decreased dramatically immediately after relationship. One of the big changes [that occurred] was that we were long distance [for the majority of our relationship], which meant we would see each other every couple of months.

And then after relationship, of course, we started living with each other. It felt like I wanted to have sex so much more and [that he wanted it] a lot less. I think while [we dated], sex was more stressful to me because of [my] religious beliefs, and so I felt more relaxed about it after relationship, and he became distant from it.

When I [would try] to talk about it, he didn't think anything was wrong and we would fight about that for years. But over the years, I had to understand that for him, sex meant having good quality sex on a less frequent basis.

Now after 10 years of relationship and two kids later, we're at a good place with it. I think one to two times a month is good for both us. Also, it helps that we know exactly what each of us like. I think that's an important place to get in your relationship as well."

—Woman, 32, married 10 years

God made sex so you'd know complete acceptance. In a group of 5 kids, were you ever the kid who didn't get paired? Exclusion happens to adults, too. We try to not worry about little slights, like not being asked out to lunch with the rest of your co-workers, but they still happen.

When you and your spouse are enjoying a moment of deep connection, you are completely accepted and accepting.

This is how God completely accepts you, "Accept one another, then, just as Christ accepted you, in order to bring praise to God," Romans 15:7.

> *"I was egotistical enough to believe that I could get him over his erectile dysfunction with my oral skills."*

22

"[The first time I was in a sexless relationship,] I had a boyfriend who had erectile dysfunction (E.D.). I was egotistical enough to believe I could get him over it with my oral skills. But I tried and failed. This was pre-Viagra time. (And before the term "E.D." was common currency.)

After a number of failures, we gave up trying. At first, he tried to satisfy my needs with his finger, and I had no objection in principle to being brought to orgasm with a finger rather than a tongue or penis, but he was so not into it.

Because it seemed like he was getting nothing for himself when he was taking care of my needs other than feeling like he was doing right by me, I finally told him to stop. I reverted to satisfying myself with my vibrator in the privacy of my home when I was not with him. (Although, we spent four nights together a week, we did not live together.)

The relationship lasted four years and eventually ended for reasons having nothing to do with the lack of sex.

My now significant other and I have been living together 13 years and are in our 70s, and he is four years younger than I am.

In the beginning, we had a healthy sex life, but he gradually got E.D. and then began losing his sex drive altogether. If I would have asked him to use his finger, he would have done it, but I had learned from the relationship I described above that if my bed partner is not enjoying what he's doing, it's not pleasurable for me either.

I'm better off just [using] my vibrator.

So, I am once again in a sexless (but otherwise great) relationship. I focus on all the positive aspects of the relationship and not on what's missing."

—Woman, 76, living with her partner for 13 years

Not everyone's comfortable talking about their sex life, but knowing what goes on in other people's bedrooms can help us all feel more inspired, curious, and validated in our own experiences. In HG's monthly column Sex IRL, we'll talk to real people about their sexual adventures and get as frank as possible.

Talk to enough people about it, and you'll realize there's no one definition of a "sexless relationship."

For some people, a sexless relationship is one where there is absolutely zero sexual activity. For others, doing everything but intercourse is considered a sexless relationship. In other situations, couples might have a ton of sex at the start of their relationship and then gradually peter out to having intercourse so infrequently that it feels basically sexless.

People have very different feelings about not having sex, too. For some people, it's a real source of tension in their relationship and a barrier to connection. For others, it's a conscious choice made because of personal beliefs about intimacy, and sticking to those beliefs feels empowering for them. And for some others, they make do without sex in their relationship, don't mind not having sex at all, or suffer in silence without it. And unfortunately, some people break up with their partners because they've been pushed to their limit.

Plenty of research has found a link between sexual satisfaction and relationship satisfaction. In other words, being happy with

24

your sex life usually plays a significant role in being happy with your overall relationship. That said, some studies have found individuals who don't have sex are just as happy with their lives as those who have sex all the time. Moreover, a 2015 study found adding more sexy time to a relationship beyond a certain point doesn't continue to improve one's well-being. (The sweet spot was once a week; less than that is associated with less happiness, but more often than that doesn't improve it.)

Perhaps the more important question is this: How important is sex to you in your relationship(s)? Every person will have their own unique feelings about sex, how often they want it, and how important it is them. It's okay to need what you need, and it's also okay for those needs to shift over time.

I spoke to 11 women who've been in sexless relationships to understand how they got there, how they felt about it, and what happened to their relationships without sex in the picture.

"Having a sexless relationship makes me feel more relaxed."

"I have been in a few, sexless relationships over the course of my dating history—all of which lasted less than a year. The relationships were sexless from the beginning mainly because I feel like I enjoy the aspect of feeling close and intimate with someone I love through sex more than the physical act itself.

From what I've experienced, sex for me is quite painful and uncomfortable. With almost every man I've ever dated, I feel like the pressure for sex is always looming overhead, but I personally don't feel sexually attracted to a man until I've gotten to know him better a few months in.

I hold out because I feel like allowing a man to have sex with me would make me vulnerable, powerless and worthless in

25

front of him afterwards. I have slept with men that have woken up the next morning completely cold and unfazed while I'm fighting back an emotional breakdown. Having a sexless relationship makes me feel more relaxed, in control and less pressured. A few men tried to change my mind, but I made it clear I didn't want to have sex. We even went as far as almost having sex with clothes on, but I insisted we not go beyond that.

This way, I don't feel like I've lost something the same way I would have sleeping with a man who I feel didn't deserve me. However, I know I will be ready to have sex with someone when I find myself falling for him, and I know he will love and accept all of me for me."

—Woman, 27, in various year-long sexless relationships

God made sex so we could understand yearning. When we are young and invincible and full of raging hormones, was the soft quiet yearning for spiritual goodness outshouted by physical realities? For some, ears aren't tuned in to the subtler cues of Christ. God gave us the physical yearning to help us understand spiritual desire.

Through experience and hopefully maturity, you see that the physical world never truly satiates the hunger. You thought it was hunger for food or sex or even human connection that you desired. But really, the hunger was placed there by God and only connecting with God and working toward his purpose in our life will we find a glimpse of satisfaction or completeness.

God placed eternity in our hearts to help us know and desire something far higher than this earth (Eccl. 3:11).

"Yes, Lord, your name and renown are the desire of our hearts. My soul yearns for you in the night; in the morning, my spirit longs for you…" Isaiah 26:8&9.

"All night long on my bed I looked for the one my heart loves; I looked for him but did not find him…I will search for the one my heart loves…. when I found the one my heart loves. I held him and would not let him go…" Song of Solomon 3:1&4.
"It was a conscious decision made on both of our behalves."

"I was with my person for a duration of about two years or so (if not more). This relationship was not a sexless one at first, but did become sexless over time, and it was a conscious decision made on both of our behalves per the Spiritual calling on my person's life. And although we faced a lot of sexual tension and challenges, we were happy to be accomplishing our goal and felt guilt-free once we eliminated all sexual intimacy. (We also became engaged.)

The abrupt downfall of this relationship took place when he allowed himself to become sexually active with another woman and later had to announce her pregnancy to me. I then cut off the engagement and decided it was best for me to go my own way in order to regroup, heal and continue to stay on my Godly path. I felt it was unfair to me when I was trying so diligently to do things God's way, along with saving myself sexually for my future husband (which was him) while he, in turn, not only broke his agreement to God first, but to me, too."

—Woman, 49, together with her partner for 2+ years

"Somehow my husband's interest in sex decreased dramatically immediately after relationship."

27

"So, in the early years of my relationship, we had a lot of issues with [not having sex]. Somehow my husband's interest in sex decreased dramatically immediately after relationship. One of the big changes [that occurred] was that we were long distance [for the majority of our relationship], which meant we would see each other every couple of months. And then after relationship, of course, we started living with each other.

It felt like I wanted to have sex so much more and [that he wanted it] a lot less. I think while [we dated], sex was more stressful to me because of [my] religious beliefs, and so I felt more relaxed about it after relationship, and he became distant from it.

When I [would try] to talk about it, he didn't think anything was wrong and we would fight about that for years. But over the years, I had to understand that for him, sex meant having good quality sex on a less frequent basis.

Now after 10 years of relationship and two kids later, we're at a good place with it. I think one to two times a month is good for both us. Also, it helps that we know exactly what each of us like. I think that's an important place to get in your relationship as well."

—Woman, 32, married 10 years

God made sex to help us stretch the borders of our life. The most vulnerable place in the world is in the middle of your relationship bed, naked with your spouse. It is in this most vulnerable place that we have tremendous power. We can nurture or we can destroy with the inflection of voice and one word.

Offering grace when you've been wronged or trying to please your spouse in a new way, both will stretch you. The stretch will allow more room in your heart for love.

"I was egotistical enough to believe that I could get him over his erectile dysfunction with my oral skills."

"[The first time I was in a sexless relationship,] I had a boyfriend who had erectile dysfunction (E.D.). I was egotistical enough to believe I could get him over it with my oral skills. But I tried and failed. This was pre-Viagra time. (And before the term "E.D." was common currency.)

After a number of failures, we gave up trying. At first, he tried to satisfy my needs with his finger, and I had no objection in principle to being brought to orgasm with a finger rather than a tongue or penis, but he was so not into it.

Because it seemed like he was getting nothing for himself when he was taking care of my needs other than feeling like he was doing right by me, I finally told him to stop. I reverted to satisfying myself with my vibrator in the privacy of my home when I was not with him. (Although, we spent four nights together a week, we did not live together.)

The relationship lasted four years and eventually ended for reasons having nothing to do with the lack of sex.

My now significant other and I have been living together 13 years and are in our 70s, and he is four years younger than I am. In the beginning, we had a healthy sex life, but he gradually got E.D. and then began losing his sex drive altogether.

If I would have asked him to use his finger, he would have done it, but I had learned from the relationship I described above that if my bed partner is not enjoying what he's doing, it's not pleasurable for me either. I'm better off just [using] my vibrator.

So, I am once again in a sexless (but otherwise great) relationship. I focus on all the positive aspects of the relationship and not on what's missing."

—*Woman, 76, living with her partner for 13 years*

God made sex so we'd have a way to extend grace. Who of us hasn't been tainted by sexual pollution before relationship or during? If not that, who hasn't transgressed through something like discord, selfish ambition, jealousy, fits of rage, dissension (Galatians 5:20). Some of those transgressions were against your spouse.

If our relationships are mirroring Christ and the church. Then, relationship is fertile field to cultivate grace. When my heart is hurt or I've hurt his, we have to reach a place of compassion, empathy, and forgiveness.

"There were so many excuses and declines that I stopped asking."

 "[Being in a sexless relationship] was a huge challenge for me. I also let my own personal solo sexual relationship die along with it. At first, we would laugh about it, but then other issues unfolded because of this happening. It just got weirder as time passed on and became the elephant in the room.

As time moved on, evidence of an unhealthy codependent relationship surfaced and I decided it was time for me to end the relationship. The ending of the relationship [was caused by many reasons]—not just [because of the lack of] sex.

[The marriage] slowly became sexless over the span of about six years. After a few years of marriage, sexual intimacy declined to about once a month, then a few times a year to nothing at all. My invitations were declined regularly. It developed to the point where there were so many excuses and declines that I stopped asking. Even cuddling or love intimacy declined to nearly no physical connection as well during the last five years of marriage.

Being in a sexless relationship was confusing and disappointing [for me]. But being sexless with my husband wasn't my choice. It hurt and I was confused as to why he was rejecting me.

I learned later it actually had nothing to do with me. Looking back, it was a gift in the end because it was one of several messages [that indicated] we were more friends than romantic partners. Other evidences of being in an unhealthy relationship unfolded as well. All of these cues led me to a divorce by my choice."

—*Woman, 46, sexless for the last five years of a 12-year marriage*

God made sex so you could quit pretending. The goal of sexual intimacy is intimacy. Intimacy is knowing someone deeply, warts and insecurities and all. The only way to achieve intimacy is to quit pretending.

We are naked physically in the marriage bed.

We should unclothe emotionally, too. No secrets.

"Adam and his wife were both naked, and they felt no shame," Genesis 2:25.

"The emotional connection created through physical connections is difficult to replicate."

"Because of physical limitations, my husband has never been able to have sex with me. Our marriage has otherwise been affectionate, but it didn't include alternatives to sex that most people suggest. My husband had such discomfort and shame around his inability to perform that he essentially closed the bedroom door permanently.

For a long time, I was able to cope with it–I've had plenty of bad sex in the past, and plenty of bad relationships that had good sex and nothing more–and being married to a good man and having an otherwise healthy connection was acceptable to me.

However, as time went on, I realized that the emotional connection created through physical connections is difficult to replicate. And during the times when a marriage naturally drifts apart, we didn't have sex as a way to reconnect.

I think over time, it made it harder and harder to stay emotionally close. Now our relationship lacks both emotional and physical intimacy, and divorce is seriously crossing my mind for the first time.

I also didn't anticipate the toll it would take on my self-image. While I understand that our situation stems completely from his physical limitations, after years of not being desired, I started to feel invisible. I struggle with this all the time, and it casts a shadow over the prospect of dating again."

—Woman, 40s, together with her husband for 12 years

Not everyone's comfortable talking about their sex life, but knowing what goes on in other people's bedrooms can help us all feel more inspired, curious, and validated in our own experiences. In HG's monthly column Sex IRL, we'll talk to real people about their sexual adventures and get as frank as possible.

Talk to enough people about it, and you'll realize there's no one definition of a "sexless relationship."

For some people, a sexless relationship is one where there is absolutely zero sexual activity. For others, doing everything but intercourse is considered a sexless relationship. In other situations, couples might have a ton of sex at the start of their relationship and then gradually peter out to having intercourse so infrequently that it feels basically sexless.

People have very different feelings about not having sex, too.

For some people, it's a real source of tension in their relationship and a barrier to connection. For others, it's a conscious choice made because of personal beliefs about intimacy, and sticking to those beliefs feels empowering for them. And for some others, they make do without sex in their relationship, don't mind not having sex at all, or suffer in silence without it. And unfortunately, some people break up with their partners because they've been pushed to their limit.

IN 365 DAYS

It doesn't take a whole lot of life experience to fully embrace the fact that God's ways are higher than our ways (Is. 55:9). Sexual intimacy is a place where we will never quite know why he created what he did. It's powerful. It's visceral. It's spiritual. It's mystifying.

When you've been a part of Godly sexuality and have a strong relationship bed, you never want to dabble in the scheme of Satan again and his counterfeit intimacy. Experiencing godly sexual intimacy helps you have a higher understanding for protecting that relationship.

God made sex really good because there are enough bad things in the world. The minutes spent in your "verdant bed" are important minutes. Godly sexual intimacy is a place where your relationship is building a fortress against the enemy who loves to distort every one of God's good gifts.

The comfort of sexual intimacy, the vision, the acceptance, all of this list counters the messages we are bombarded with by the Prince of Darkness.

Relationship isn't easy and everyone of us heard the saying 'relationship is work' at least once. And yes, once the honeymoon stage is over, it's not so easy to maintain a fulfilling and wholesome relationship, but there must be certain red flags that obviously show that the relationship isn't working the way it should be.

If so, what are those red flags? Is lack of romance and intimacy a red flag? What about a passive-aggressive excel spreadsheet displaying all of the days you refused to sleep with your partner?

There are varying definitions of a sexless relationship or sexless relationship: no sex in the past year, no sex in the past six months or sex 10 or fewer times a year. According to one study, approximately 15 percent of married couples are sexless: Spouses haven't had sex with each other in the past six months to one year.

I Was in a sexless relationship, I have debated admitting this publicly, but my story feels different than the narrative advanced by our patriarchal society. Why? Because I was the one begging for sex from an uninterested female partner. Sex 10 times a year would have been 10 times more than what I was having.

This topic comes up a lot when I was out with my friends. I'm frequently asked about the "right number" of times to have sex a month. The answer is that there isn't one. If both people are truly happy, then it's a healthy sex life.

I understand the confusion about frequency. Messaging around sex is everywhere: It's used to sell almost everything, and news articles remind us that various hormones and neurotransmitters may spike in response to having sex.

Yet a single hormone surge does not a rewarding relationship make, and virtually no one has studied the hormonal impact, on a relationship, of grocery shopping, making dinner or doing the dishes. If a couple doesn't have sex but they both feel satisfied, then there is no problem. The issue is when there's a mismatch in desire.

Of course, libido ebbs and flows, and there will be times when one partner is temporarily uninterested. Back in 1999, I was home with two premature infants, both on oxygen and attached to monitors that constantly chirped with alarms.

Looking back on my relationship, the frequency of sex dropped off quickly. I told myself it would get better because there were other positives. I falsely assumed that women have higher libidos, so clearly this was temporary.

Pro tip: Nothing in a relationship ever gets better on its own. You might as well ask the ingredients in your pantry to bake themselves into a cake.

I was embarrassed when my attempts at rekindling the magic — things like sleeping naked or trying to schedule date night sex.

I started to circuitously ask friends if they ever felt similarly rejected. The answer was "Not really." One who was going through an especially acrimonious divorce told me that he and his future ex still occasionally had wild sex. People have needs, after all.

The fact that people who hated each other were having more sex than me did not make me feel better. Not at all.

Eventually I decided that sympathy sex once or twice a year was far worse than no sex. I worried that no intervention would be sustainable, and the time not addressing the issue had simply taken its toll. We were terribly mismatched sexually, and it wasn't something that she was interested in addressing.

My experience led me to listen differently to men speaking about their sex lives with women, whether in on the radio or in my personal life. There are spaces between words that tell entire stories. When I ask someone about his sex life and there is a pause or a generic "O.K.," I say, "You know, the libido issue is often with the woman."

I say this to friends, acquaintances and even people I barely know on airplane. The responses from men are so similar that I could script it. A pause, then relief that it's not just them, followed quickly by the desire to hear more. Many tell me intimate details, so glad to have someone in whom they can confide.

Libido can be affected by a number of things, including depression, medication, stress, health, affairs, previous sexual trauma, pornography, pain with sex and relationship dissatisfaction (having sex while going through an ugly divorce is probably an outlier). Erectile dysfunction is a factor for some women, especially over the age of 45. There is also the possibility that one partner in a heterosexual relationship is gay.

New love is intoxicating, and I'm not being metaphorical.

A functional MRI study suggests that new love activates the reward centers of the brain and, like opioids, increases pain tolerance. I wonder how much the drug that is new love affects libido? If some women and men are simply on a lower libido spectrum in everyday life, might they revert to that once this "love drug" subsides, leaving those with a higher libido frustrated?

I want men to know that if they are on the wanting end for sex, they are not alone. If you love the person you're with, then the sooner you speak up, the better. You can try what I did — sleeping naked and scheduling sex — because the more you have sex, the more you may want to have it, if you're doing it right and it feels good. However, if things are not changing in the way you want, you may need help from a couple's counselor, a sex therapist, a clinical psychologist or a medical doctor, depending on the situation.

Waiting until months or even years have passed can weaponized the bedroom. It will add so much more complexity because resentment compounds like a high-interest credit card.

Sexuality and relationships are complex, and there are no easy answers. It's not good or bad to have a high, a medium or a low libido. You like what you like, but if you don't speak up about what you want, you can't expect the other person to know.

Our society seems almost built on the erroneous idea that all men want sex all the time, so I imagine it would be hard for men to admit to a lower libido, even anonymously. I have lied about my weight on many forms. That doesn't make me a broken person; it just proves that a cloak of invisibility doesn't hide you from yourself.

The most damaging lies are the ones we tell ourselves. Physical intimacy is commonly what makes a romantic relationship more than just a platonic friendship. Some couples slip into a pattern or habit of letting the physical part of their relationship fall by the wayside. Others had little to no sex from the start.

Many couples experience a drop-off in sex and physical intimacy within the first few years of relationship, particularly if kids come into the picture. However, the complete loss of physical intimacy that once was a part of the relationship often signals a problem that needs to be addressed.

Without the physical intimacy that differentiates a romantic partnership from a platonic one, married couples can become more-or-less roommates. If both partners are OK with this type of relationship, it doesn't call for concern. But often, one or both partners become frustrated or hurt by the loss of physical intimacy and sex.

GOD MADE SEX

To extend the meaning of marriage beyond best friends, buddies, or friends with benefits. Marriage is more than just living under the same roof. Marriage is more than a legality so that you can jointly file taxes. He creates a new unit when you pledge yourselves to each other.

"Did he not make them one, with a portion of the Spirit in their union?" Malachi 2:15.

God glues a husband and wife together. In Mark 10:7, "For this cause shall a man leave his father and mother, and cleave to his wife..." The word cleave is translated from the Greek word, proskollao. Its essence means to join as if glued together.

This covenant is sealed with more than a kiss. It's sealed with conjugal love. Sexual intimacy, which creates one flesh, reflecting the spiritual intimacy we should seek with God.

Love making not only seals the covenant, but each time you make love your body also creates silken emotional bonds, soft and oh so very strong. God created sexual intimacy in a way that it releases chemicals in our brains that create trust and companionship.

God made sex for the seasons of life. Song of Solomon 2:11-12, "See! The winter is past; the rains are over and gone. Flowers appear on the earth; the season of singing has come; the cooing of doves is heard in our land."

Remember Abraham and Sarah?

Remember John and Elizabeth? Both couples had babies in their elder years by God's miracle. Sexual intimacy isn't only

39

for the young. It's for all seasons of marriage. It tethers husband and wife to the sacred moments of years of marriage.

As experiences of life bring wisdom and bodies evolve with time, sexual intimacy is the act that connects the two of you to the moments of your young marriage, when life was full of sweet anticipation.

Sex is a little like time travel.

"It was a conscious decision made on both of our behalves."

"I was with my person for a duration of about two years or so (if not more). This relationship was not a sexless one at first, but did become sexless over time, and it was a conscious decision made on both of our behalves per the Spiritual calling on my person's life. And although we faced a lot of sexual tension and challenges, we were happy to be accomplishing our goal and felt guilt-free once we eliminated all sexual intimacy. (We also became engaged.)

The abrupt downfall of this relationship took place when he allowed himself to become sexually active with another woman and later had to announce her pregnancy to me.

I then cut off the engagement and decided it was best for me to go my own way in order to regroup, heal and continue to stay on my Godly path. I felt it was unfair to me when I was trying so diligently to do things God's way, along with saving myself sexually for my future husband (which was him) while he, in turn, not only broke his agreement to God first, but to me, too."

—*Woman, 49, together with her partner for 2+ years*

God made sex to help us lighten up. Sexual intimacy isn't very dignified. The other day, I answered someone over lunch with a mouth-full of food and it was somebody I wanted to impress. I was embarrassed and realized that I'm not always that classy. My embarrassment lingers.

But, it is what it is. That's how it is with sexual intimacy. It is what it is. A bit gooshy, a bit contorted, a bit unpredictable, a bit unmannerly. The marriage bed is a place to impress with love, not impress with Emily Post etiquette.

There's another good thing about lightening up before you meet in the bedroom, it can lead to sexual desire.

"Somehow my husband's interest in sex decreased dramatically immediately after marriage."

"So, in the early years of my marriage, we had a lot of issues with [not having sex]. Somehow my husband's interest in sex decreased dramatically immediately after marriage.

One of the big changes [that occurred] was that we were long distance [for the majority of our relationship], which meant we would see each other every couple of months. And then after marriage, of course, we started living with each other.

It felt like I wanted to have sex so much more and [that he wanted it] a lot less. I think while [we dated], sex was more stressful to me because of [my] religious beliefs, and so I felt more relaxed about it after marriage, and he became distant from it.

When I [would try] to talk about it, he didn't think anything was wrong and we would fight about that for years. But over the

41

years, I had to understand that for him, sex meant having good quality sex on a less frequent basis.

Now after 10 years of marriage and two kids later, we're at a good place with it. I think one to two times a month is good for both us. Also, it helps that we know exactly what each of us like. I think that's an important place to get in your relationship as well."

—Woman, 32, married 10 years

God made sex to give us a moment's peace. A busy life singes our joy like a hot sun. Low libido sisters, we have to pursue arousal amidst busy minds. Once we find arousal, there are a few moments of yearning to press on. During the moments of yearning, we can escape the hot sun of busyness and rest, to "delight to sit in his shade," (Song of Solomon 2:3), to savor a moment's peace.

For those brief moments of peace, "You are a garden fountain, a well of flowing water streaming down from Lebanon," Song of Solomon 4:15.

"I was egotistical enough to believe that I could get him over his erectile dysfunction with my oral skills."

"[The first time I was in a sexless relationship,] I had a boyfriend who had erectile dysfunction (E.D.). I was egotistical enough to believe I could get him over it with my oral skills. But I tried and failed. This was pre-Viagra time. (And before the term "E.D." was common currency.) After a number of failures, we gave up trying.

At first, he tried to satisfy my needs with his finger, and I had no objection in principle to being brought to orgasm with a finger rather than a tongue or penis, but he was so not into it.

Because it seemed like he was getting nothing for himself when he was taking care of my needs other than feeling like he was doing right by me, I finally told him to stop. I reverted to satisfying myself with my vibrator in the privacy of my home when I was not with him. (Although, we spent four nights together a week, we did not live together.)

The relationship lasted four years and eventually ended for reasons having nothing to do with the lack of sex.

My now significant other and I have been living together 19 years and are in our 70s, and he is four years younger than I am. In the beginning, we had a healthy sex life, but he gradually got E.D. and then began losing his sex drive altogether.

If I would have asked him to use his finger, he would have done it, but I had learned from the relationship I described above that if my bed partner is not enjoying what he's doing, it's not pleasurable for me either. I'm better off just [using] my vibrator.

So, I am once again in a sexless (but otherwise great) relationship. I focus on all the positive aspects of the relationship and not on what's missing."

—Woman, 76, living with her partner for 19 years

God made sexual fulfillment of equal value for the husband and wife. "The husband should fulfill his marital duty to his wife, and likewise the wife to her husband.

The wife does not have authority over her own body, but the husband. Likewise, the husband does not have authority over his own body, but the wife.

Do not deprive one another, except by mutual consent for a limited time, so you may devote yourselves to prayer. Then come together again, so that Satan will not tempt you through your lack of self-control," 1 Corinthians 7:3-5.

Get that? The husband's sex drive is not more important than the wife's. The wife's sex drive is not more important than the husband's.

In other words, neither spouse's sexual need in a marriage trumps the other. One does not get the privilege of saying, "No," all the time and the other doesn't get the privilege of demanding a, "Yes," all the time.

You figure out a happy common ground. And yes, I think marital duty includes helping each other feel fully satisfied. Don't deprive one another.

If you're a low drive spouse, I completely understand how this seems hard. But, you know what? You knew going in that sex was meant to be a common practice in your weekly marital life. Besides, you couldn't wait to hop in the sack in the newlywed days, right? That hotness can be re-discovered, honest!

"There were so many excuses and declines that I stopped asking."

"[Being in a sexless relationship] was a huge challenge for me. I also let my own personal solo sexual relationship die along with it. At first, we would laugh about it, but then other issues unfolded because of this happening. It just got weirder as time passed on and became the elephant in the room.

As time moved on, evidence of an unhealthy codependent relationship surfaced and I decided it was time for me to end the marriage. The ending of the marriage [was caused by many reasons]—not just [because of the lack of] sex.

[The marriage] slowly became sexless over the span of about six years. After a few years of marriage, sexual intimacy declined to about once a month, then a few times a year to nothing at all. My invitations were declined regularly.

It developed to the point where there were so many excuses and declines that I stopped asking. Even cuddling or love intimacy declined to nearly no physical connection as well during the last five years of marriage.

Being in a sexless relationship was confusing and disappointing [for me]. But being sexless with my husband wasn't my choice. It hurt and I was confused as to why he was rejecting me.

I learned later it actually had nothing to do with me.

Looking back, it was a gift in the end because it was one of several messages [that indicated] we were more friends than romantic partners. Other evidences of being in an unhealthy relationship unfolded as well. All of these cues led me to a divorce by my choice."

—*Woman, 52, sexless for the last five years of a 29-year marriage*

God made sex as playdates for mates. Tired of adulating? Fine. Take your middle school mind into the bedroom and have some fun. When there is an accidental puffing or someone falls off the bed, all the better for your inner middle schooler.

Remember when you were in middle school and everything had a sexual connotation because adolescent hormones were firing? Well, read this next verse with your adolescent attitude and think of your spouse.

"I went down to the grove of nut trees to look at the new growth in the valley, to see if the vines had budded or the pomegranates were in bloom." Song of Solomon 6:11.

"He confessed that he felt turned off by my weight."

"[Our relationship] became sexless over time [during the] last four years of the relationship. It happened after my depression happened, which lasted about three years and, as he mentioned, because we gained weight.

It was frustrating for me. I tried to enjoy my own company and even masturbation did not feel like enough at the time. I felt neglected and abandoned. I felt like he did make a few attempts [to improve the situation], but I felt like I tried more.

But it became this weird back and forth ... [During] days I was in the mood and I tried [to have sex with him], he rejected me. And on times he wanted [to have sex], since I felt rejected, I did decline too because I wasn't in the mood to feel rejected again.

It became worse when he allowed his best guy friend to live with us in the house. It got so bad that one night after watching HBO's True Blood, I was aroused by some of the sexy scenes that I wanted to play flirty with him and entice him for us to be intimate. However, he said, "Here we go again. I already told you I'm not in the mood.

46

My best friend is next door (in the living room)." This statement took the cake for me to begin to switch and transition; it was time to let him go. I told him, "You've been telling me that story even before he got here. If you don't want me, just say it."

That is when he said that we were both overweight, and he feels he's not turned on because he could not see his thing. In addition, he confessed that he felt turned off by my weight and the condition the house was in during my depressive years.

He said he felt neglected by me then and because he had to work and order food for us since I didn't cook."

—*Woman, 38, sexless for the last four years of a 17-year relationship*

> *"The emotional connection created through physical connections is difficult to replicate."*

"Because of physical limitations, my husband has never been able to have sex with me. Our marriage has otherwise been affectionate, but it didn't include alternatives to sex that most people suggest. My husband had such discomfort and shame around his inability to perform that he essentially closed the bedroom door permanently.

For a long time, I was able to cope with it–I've had plenty of bad sex in the past, and plenty of bad relationships that had good sex and nothing more–and being married to a good man and having an otherwise healthy connection was acceptable to me.

However, as time went on, I realized that the emotional connection created through physical connections is difficult to replicate. And during the times when a marriage naturally drifts apart, we didn't have sex as a way to reconnect.

I think over time, it made it harder and harder to stay emotionally close. Now our relationship lacks both emotional and physical intimacy, and divorce is seriously crossing my mind for the first time.

I also didn't anticipate the toll it would take on my self-image. While I understand that our situation stems completely from his physical limitations, after years of not being desired, I started to feel invisible. I struggle with this all the time, and it casts a shadow over the prospect of dating again."

—*Woman, 40s, together with her husband for 16 years*

God made sex messy so we remember that life is messy. Well, who could really forget that life is messy? Some seasons are better than others, but life is hard. Yes, you can take measures to contain the mess in life and in the bedroom. But, that just stifles the mood. Roll with it. Let God be in control, in your life and in the bedroom.

Chances are your spouse doesn't care as much as you about the mess. Embrace the mess, those fluids contain the divine spark! Maybe think of it as, "Liquid Awesome!"

"I later found out he had been sleeping with his best friend for months."

"I was in a sexless relationship for three years. It wasn't my choice to be sexless, it was his. He said that we should be saving sex for marriage, and that was that. We did everything but sex, which really messed with me. It put the concept of sex on a pedestal, and made me want it more but also, made me disgusted by it. I also had this false sense of "holier-than-though," because I felt like I was "better" or more "disciplined" for not having sex—at least that's how I justified it. We broke up after three years because he wasn't into me anymore.

I later found out he had been sleeping with his best friend for months, and worse, that everyone but me knew. That really, really messed with me. I went from feeling holier-then-thou to feeling like I wasn't woman enough for him or that I wasn't attractive, just not enough. It took me a long time to digest and get over what happened. It also changed how I viewed sex.

It wasn't until I read the book Come as You Are that I fully understood and resolved those feelings of inadequacy."

—Woman, 32, together with her partner for 7 years

God made sex to help us know him in the most intimate way.

Just as God uses communion and baptism to represent spiritual meaning, have you ever thought that sexual intimacy could mirror the type of intimate relationship God wants to have with us?

In the way that Adam knew Eve, God wants to know us. Why would I make such a bold statement? The key is a little Hebrew word, Yada. Yada is the Hebrew word for "intimately know," to know someone as intimately as a lover.

"Be still and know [yada] that I am God," Psalm 46:10.

"Oh, Lord, thou hast searched me and thou know [yada] me," Psalm 139:1.

"We've started to get better."
"My husband and I have been together for 22 years and have been sexless for most of our marriage, including a stint where

we went less than a week shy of a calendar year. Both of us had histories of being sexually abused, him when he was quite young and me during my late teens to early twenties.

We did okay with regular sex when we were dating, but within months of the honeymoon, we were in marriage counseling because it was already apparent that we were heading toward a sexless marriage.

Being young, physically healthy, and happily married while lacking physical intimacy is fraught with problems. People just assume you're having sex very often and would make comments that were so wildly inappropriate even if we HAD been having sex often, but stung a lot when I knew we weren't. The kicker is that we're not bad at sex.

We're actually really good at sex.

We can orgasm simultaneously in various positions without clitoral stimulation, which is like going Easter egg hunting and finding a Faberge instead. But when that lone simultaneous beautiful orgasm happens once or twice or thrice annually, that is as much a cruelty as it is a blessing. How can a couple be this good in bed together, so good at satisfying each other in the moment, and yet so bad at connecting toward even kissing?

Without warning or particular provocation, just in the past eight or nine months, we've started to get better. Recently, we even had sex twice within two weeks. It's been eight years, if not more, since that happened. I can't say whether or not being sexless is residing or if we're just on a temporary hiatus. I'm happy to have these times for now, though."

—*Woman, 34, together with her partner for 18 years*

50

God designed the orgasm, O Lord! How manifold thy works! (Psalm 104:24) All things were created by God (Col. 1:16).

God delights in his creation (Zephaniah 3:17).

God delights to give his creation good gifts (James 1:17).

When he created orgasm (one of those good gifts), God probably said with a wink, "Oh, they're going to like this!"

Orgasm is encouraged and if you've never experienced orgasm, give yourself permission to pursue it with research. And maybe, just maybe, he created the ultimate moment in sexual intimacy to mirror the ecstasy we will feel when glorifying him in his presence.

Maybe the moment of ecstasy is just the preview.

"I'm empowering myself to find the sex I've been praying for."

"I'm a clergy woman in a sexless marriage. For me, that means there is no sexual intercourse. In fact, I hate to admit that our marriage was never consummated. We went to pre-marital counseling. We talked about sex, especially given our 14-year age difference. He is 14-years my senior. We agreed that if there were challenges around sex, he would get whatever assistance, Viagra. However, years into the marriage, he never got the prescription filled.

It wasn't a personal choice. I resulted to self-satisfaction with B.O.B., aka my battery-operated boyfriend. It has been humiliating, embarrassing, and a self-esteem robber. I often wonder and I've even asked what's wrong with me?

I've asked, why he isn't attracted to me? Until finally, I've stopped asking.

The tensions have impacted our marriage. So much so, I've finally resolved to file for divorce. This year, I will be celebrating my 46th birthday. I want to extricate myself from this sexless and ultimately, loveless union so I can be available to meet someone new.

As a clergy woman, I've prayed. However, I believe God can only do so much. We have a part to play in getting our prayers answered. He's refused to exercise options available to him. But I'm empowering myself to find the sex I've been praying for.

—Woman, 44, together with her partner for four years

WHY THE SEX STOP?

People stop for a variety of reasons. Common reasons are a lack of desire, postpartum depression, frequent marital conflict, or a recent marital crisis or personal crisis that has impacted the client. When couples begin noticing a lack of sexual contact in their relationship, they should see that as a crucial time to address it directly and discern what is causing the change.

Top reasons for not putting out:

1- Low or non-existent sex drive
2- Relationship issues
3- Lack of love and closeness
4- Unresolved trauma in one or both partners' past
5- Chronic Illness or medical reasons
6- Sexual dysfunction or sexual pain
7- Childcare stresses or family dynamics
8- Lack of sexual desire or attraction
9- Hormonal imbalance
10- Mental health issues

LOW SEX DRIVE
Many people simply have a low sex drive. Some folks have never had much interest in sexual activity, while others experience changes in drive due to physical or mental health issues. An individual's sex drive is also bound to hamper if he or she initiates sex with a partner and is repeatedly turned down.

If you have no interest in sex with your partner, but you're interested in sex with others, the issue is likely not drive, but a problem within the marriage-perhaps one or more of the issues that we'll discuss in the rest of this section.

LACK OF EMOTIONAL CONNECTION

When a marriage lacks emotional connection, the couple's sex life tends to become nonexistent over time. Sexual intimacy is impossible to maintain when partners don't feel emotionally connected. This emotional void often becomes damaging to a marriage, as couples feel distant from each other and often stop having sex altogether.

Poor Communication Regarding Needs. Even within a marriage, many individuals don't know how to talk about sex. Poor communication can result in unsatisfying sex or lack of sexual intimacy. A healthy sex life requires open communication, where partners voices their needs and desires and practice active listening.

MEDICAL PROBLEMS

A wide range of medical issues can affect libido and impede the enjoyment of sexual experiences. High blood pressure, diabetes, medications, vitamin deficiencies, hormonal problems, smoking, obesity, and thyroid dysfunction are just a few physical problems that can contribute.

We've mentioned already – and we'll mention again – that there are mental and emotional health experts that can help you have a healthy sex life.

However, you should also bring your problems up with your regular healthcare provider. It could be a symptom of life factors that could endanger more than just your sex life.

DISABILITY

Some disabilities may cause sexual dysfunction. In the case that intercourse isn't possible, couples may be able to engage in other sexual activities that meet both partners' needs and desires.

MENTAL HEALTH ISSUES
Mental health conditions, such as depression and anxiety can keep one or both partners from maintaining a sex life that meets both their needs and desires. Individuals going through a major mental health condition may struggle to find the energy for sexual activity, and in some cases, the spouse may take on a caretaking role, which can put a damper on a couple's intimate relationship.

Antidepressant medications can cause erectile dysfunction and vaginal dryness, while anti-anxiety medications can lessen excitement.

If you think that a medication – whether for mental and emotional health or other conditions – is causing the problem, bring it up with the prescribing physician. He or she may be able to put you on a different medication or adjust your dose to try to minimize side effects.

CHILDREN
Having children can hamper a couple's sex life for a multitude of reasons. Women experience changes in their bodies during pregnancy. Hormones get out of their normal balance, and breastfeeding causes prolactin levels to soar, causing vaginal thinning and dryness, which can make sex uncomfortable or even painful. Raising children also takes a lot of energy.

Many parents experience a variety of stress-related mental and physical health problems that can decrease their desire for sex. Plus, if you're worried about having sex when your children are awaking or in the house, it can really limit your windows of opportunity.

AGE-RELATED FACTORS

As we age, our bodies go through a series of changes. Women often experience a drop-in estrogen, while low testosterone can be a problem for both men and women. Older men are more likely to experience erectile dysfunction, while some women experience vaginal dryness. While our energy levels tend to decrease as we age, there is good news: People over 60 tend to have more sexual confidence than they did earlier in life.

Still, coping with a sexless marriage can be difficult at any age. particular if other life factors like health issues are also making things difficult.

UNRESOLVED ANGER

Unresolved anger may be the reason you and your partner aren't having sex. In some cases, sexless marriages end in divorce, with couples citing sexual problems as a major contributor. In actuality, unresolved anger and resentment may have led to the lack of sex.

WHEN YOU STOP HAVE SEX YOUR BODY PAYS

MENTAL HEALTH
Some people equate having a sex life with their self-worth. Although this is not the case, they may feel more anxious and depressed if they go a long period of time without having sex. It's important to remember that your value does not come from having sex with other people.

LIBIDO
Surprisingly, going a long time without having sex can make you lose interest in sex altogether. The more you have sex, the more you want to have sex. Regular sex boosts your libido.

YOU GET MORE STRESSED OUT
A great night of lovemaking can make literally everything else in the world feel better. Even if your boss won't stop breathing down your neck, or if you're under a bunch of deadlines, you're consistently getting laid, so all of that stuff seems super manageable.

Apparently, there's a scientific reason for that. Neuroscientist during orgasm, "endorphins are released that can help to improve your mood." "So, if you tend to use sex as a way of coping with stress, a dry spell can be doubly frustrating."

YOU DON'T SLEEP AS WELL
We know from numerous studies that sleep is directly related to stress. When you're stressed, you don't tend to get quality sleep. (This creates a vicious cycle because when you don't sleep, you end up getting more stressed.) Sex helps your de-stress by releasing numerous hormones and neurotransmitters.

Phil Stieg M.D., Ph.D., neurosurgeon-in-chief at New York-Presbyterian Weill Cornell Medical Center and host of the This

Is Your Brain podcast previously that the release of three hormones, in particular, facilitate better sleep: oxytocin; prolactin; and dopamine. "Oxytocin has a very calming effect, and as anyone who has ever tried to fall asleep while stressed out knows, being calm is the best way to prepare for sleep," he said. "Prolactin creates a sense of satisfaction, and dopamine is known as the feel-good hormone.

So, in short, when you have sex, you're less likely to be stressed, and you're more likely to sleep better.

YOUR BLOOD PRESSURE CAN SPIKE
Without sex, you may notice an increase in blood pressure. Science says that's not a coincidence. In fact, a 2006 study in the medical journal Biological Psychology found that people who were having regular sex had lower levels of blood pressure than those who weren't. This is also linked to the relationship between sex and stress.

The researchers controlled for multiple variables in the study and concluded that having sex more frequently actually improves your body's physiological response to stress. This, in turn, keeps one's blood pressure at a lower base level.

RELATIONSHIP HEALTH
For many couples, regular sexual intercourse is an important way to maintain their bond. Regular sex also often leads to *better communication*.

Generally, couples who have sex more often feel more emotionally attached and connected in comparison with those who do it less often. What happens when you don't have sex for a long time?

For some people, their relationship with their partner becomes more stressful and they stop feeling connected. Other couples aren't interested in sex or they don't find it to be an important way of connecting, preferring conversation or shared activities instead.

HEART DISEASE
A 2010 study published in the American Journal of Cardiology found that men who have sex at least twice a week almost cut their risk of heart disease in half. However, the researchers noted their findings may simply be correlational—not causal.

"Men who have frequent sex might be more likely to be in a supportive intimate relationship," they noted. "This might improve health through stress reduction and social support."

CARDIOVASCULAR HEALTH
If you do not have sex on a regular basis, you are at a higher risk of developing cardiovascular disease. In addition to being a source of exercise, sexual intercourse helps keep your estrogen and progesterone levels in balance, which can lower your risk of heart disease.

YOUR SEX RHYTHM IS OFF
You know that old expression, "if you don't use it, you lose it?" Science suggests that to a degree, that might be true. A 2008 study in the American Journal of Medicine concluded that men in their 50s, 60s, and 70s that weren't sexually active were more likely to suffer from erectile dysfunction.

This makes some sense: on an intellectual level, navigating all those arms and legs and erogenous zones can get pretty confusing, so imagine trying to navigate the core mechanics of intercourse after months and months of not having sex at all.

Luckily, there's an easy solution: even if you don't have a partner, the research suggests ejaculating regularly can help alleviate some of these effects.

IF YOU DON'T MASTURBATE, PROSTATE GOES UP

If your dry spell extends to the self-pleasure zone — i.e., if you're not masturbating at all — research says that's not healthy.

In fact, multiple studies have pointed to the conclusion that "high ejaculation frequency" (a.k.a. jerking off at least 4.6 to seven times a week) is linked to a lower risk of prostate cancer.

So, get out those baby wipes and turn on Pornhub for the sake of your own health.

VAGINAL HEALTH

Having sex after a long break can be uncomfortable. It takes longer for the female body to become aroused and produce enough lubrication to make sex easy and comfortable.

Regular sex or masturbation can keep the tissues in your vagina healthy by improving blood flow.

YOUR IMMUNE SYSTEM GETS WEAKER

Orgasms are incredibly beneficial to your immune system, as psychologists Carl Charnetski and Francis Brennan Jr. found.

They conducted a study where they asked patients who were having sex once or twice a week to provide saliva samples.

Those samples were found to contain an extremely high concentration of the common-cold busting antibody immunoglobulin, who knew that extremely close contact was a net-positive in terms of preventing illness?

YOUR DREAMS CHANGE

One of the weirdest things to change if you're not having sex is your dreams, according to the aforementioned. The nice thing is that you'll start having sex dreams and even possibly orgasming in your sleep.

YOUR SEX DRIVE MAY DISAPPEAR

Your body might actually stop asking for orgasms if you don't have any for an extended period of time, according to the aforementioned Prevention article. The lack of lust is just your body protecting itself, but masturbation is a good idea if you want to keep your sex drive at its normal level.

YOUR SELF-ESTEEM MIGHT SUFFER

Not having sex might make you feel less attractive. This might be because semen has anti-depressant qualifies — and yes, that's not just a myth.

YOUR WORK PERFORMANCE MIGHT SLIP

Most dry spells have two parts: the part where you're insanely horny and turned on by even a slightly curvaceous frying pain; and the part where you're down in the dumps and can't even be motivated to get off the couch. Apparently, that can even spill over into your employment satisfaction. An Oregon State University study found that couples with an active sex life were much happier at work.

"Maintaining a healthy relationship that includes a healthy sex life will help employees stay happy and engaged in their work, which benefits the employees and the organizations they work for," says Keith Leavitt, an associate professor at the college.

There you go, guys: feel free to blame missing that Zoom call on not getting laid. I'm sure your boss will understand.

Does sexless marriage justify adultery?

When you married, you likely made a promise, explicitly or implicitly, that you would not cheat on your spouse. So, violating the marital agreement is not justified under any condition.

With that said, spouses typically promise when they marry that they would tend to the needs of each person. This includes sexual needs. If one partner has stopped engaging in sex, and is unwilling to address that, they also likely violated the marital agreement.

Solving your sexless marriage with adultery is a highly risky and traumatic decision. Adultery, risks the physical and emotional health of a marriage.

What age do people stop being sexually active?

It is common knowledge that people often have sex less frequently as they age. This is particularly true between midlife and later life. This is due to a variety of factors. However, there is no set age in which people are unable or incapable of having sex.

In fact, people in the age group of 70+ are seemingly having more sex now than that same age group in the past.

Sleep disturbances are a regular part of being a new parent, in this situation a sleep disturbance tends to be characterized by difficulty sleeping even when the infant is asleep, and others have offered to care for the infant.

To survive a marriage with no sex and without cheating?

Sadly, many people have to live in a marriage where there is no sex happening. They endure this by using a variety of strategies. Some include frequent masturbation, grieving the loss of their sex life, and trying to focus more on what they are getting out the marriage rather than what they are not.

Some couples have agreed to allow exceptions to their fidelity agreement, including opening up their marriage. If this is something you are wanting to try, please consider working with a couple's counselor first as this strategy can backfire if done poorly.

Is a sexless marriage grounds for divorce?

That is an individual decision. People divorce for many reasons, and many believe their reasons justify their decision. It is problematic if your partner regularly declines having sex with you. Also, if your spouse also doesn't have any interest in changing that, then you are being faced with a very difficult problem. Living without and sexual touch or intimacy can be troubling and damaging to your health.

Before considering divorce, consider working with a sex therapist as it can help couples improve their sex lives and save their relationship.

COMMON REASONS

There are many possible reasons that a marriage may become sexless, including everything from health issues to lifestyle factors. Here's an overview of some common reasons.

HEALTH ISSUES

A person's overall physical and mental health can have a major impact on their libido and desire for physical intimacy. Health concerns and disability can also disrupt the physiological process of arousal in both sexes.

Experiencing some problems with sexual functioning is common, but if they last for more than a few months or they're causing problems for you or your partner, it's a good idea to speak with a healthcare provider.

MISMATCHED LIBIDOS

Not everyone desires the same amount of sex, and sex drive has a natural ebb and flow. When the desire for sex does not coincide, it's easy for couples to find themselves waiting to engage sexually until both partners are in the mood, which can be infrequent.

CHILDBIRTH

According to The American College of Obstetricians and Gynecologists, there isn't a defined time when someone can have sex again after childbirth, but many healthcare providers recommend waiting for at least four to six weeks (though sometimes longer) for physical recovery alone.

This timeframe of no sex typically wouldn't be long enough to be considered a true "sexless marriage," but whether someone who gave birth is mentally and emotionally ready to have sex after this point depends on the individual. The added stress of caring for an infant, body changes, tiredness, and hormonal factors can also affect a person's libido after having a child.

STRESS

Excessive stress can wreak havoc on your health, including your sex drive. The stress hormone cortisol can also play a role in lowering your libido. In addition to the physical reasons why stress lowers sex drive, the psychological effects of stress can leave you so tired, frazzled, and anxious that you simply don't have the desire or energy for sex.

COMMUNICATION ISSUES
When you are in conflict with your partner, it can be difficult to maintain physical intimacy. You might not feel like talking to your partner, let alone engaging in sexual activity.

Contributing Factors
- Conflicts and arguments
- Negative feelings
- Punitive or passive-aggressive behaviors
- Infidelity
- Power struggles
- Pornography addiction

ERECTILE DYSFUNCTION
Difficulty achieving or maintaining an erection can make it difficult to have sex for a number of reasons. While erectile dysfunction (ED) is a common problem, it can also affect a person's anxiety levels, confidence, and self-esteem. People who have symptoms of ED should always talk to a doctor, as it may be a sign of an underlying health condition.

LOW SEX DRIVE
Sometimes called hypoactive sexual desire disorder, low sex drive is an issue that both men and women may experience.

In females, a number of factors may contribute to, including menstrual cycles, the use of hormonal contraceptives, childbirth, breastfeeding, hysterectomy, and menopause.

MEDICATION SIDE EFFECTS
Many medications have sexual side effects. Some drugs that can cause sexual dysfunction include over-the-counter

decongestants, some antihistamines, antidepressants, and high blood pressure medications.

MENTAL HEALTH ISSUES
Symptoms of depression include lack of energy, loss of interest and pleasure, social withdrawal, and depressed mood—all factors that can have an effect on a person's desire for sex and physical intimacy.

HISTORY OF ABUSE
Past sexual abuse can have long-lasting effects that can influence current and future relationships. Emotional reactions such as fear and shame, post-traumatic stress, and distortions in self-perception can have a serious impact on a person's sex life.

LIFE ISSUES
There are a number of different life factors that can also play a role in how frequently people engage in sex with their partner, including:

- Aging
- Body image issues
- Boredom
- Financial problems
- Grief
- Job loss
- Tiredness

What to do if your partner is uninterested in sex

HOW TO ADDRESS THE ISSUE
The first step is recognizing that you have a low-sex or NO-SEX marriage and determining whether a lack of sex is a problem for your marriage. Whether you consider a low-sex or

NO-SEX marriage an issue is entirely up to you and your partner.

There is no right amount of sex to have in a marriage. What's more important, in many cases, is whether you still have physical and emotional intimacy with your partner and whether both you and your partner are satisfied in your marriage.

Avoid comparing your marriage to others because every relationship is unique. While you might come across statistics that make you feel like you and your partner are not having enough sex, research has found that going without sex is more common than you might think.

According to General Social Survey data from 1972 to 2004, 6% of married couples were sexually inactive over the previous year. However, it's important to note that for just younger couples (ages 18 to 49), the percentage is much lower at 1.3 to 2.5%.7

Here are some ways you can address the lack of sex in your marriage if it's a problem for you and your partner.

COMMUNICATE
Talk with your partner about the issue of low or no sex in your marriage. It may be difficult, but this communication is necessary. Even otherwise strong relationships can have problems with sex and intimacy. It isn't necessarily a sign that your marriage is weak or in trouble.

Lack of sex may simply mean that you need to talk more and carve out more time to spend together as a couple.

If you need help figuring out how to talk to your partner, consider first talking to a mental health professional or therapist for ideas about how to approach the subject. It is important to keep the conversation positive and not leave your partner feeling like they are being attacked or blamed.

Every relationship is different and you will need to work together as a couple to figure out what works for you. Don't try to live up to other people's expectations or what you think is normal. Talk about what each of you wants, needs, and expects. Then work together to make it work for both of you.

As you talk, aim to determine ways you both think you can rekindle your sex life. Making a change will only work if both of you agree to change and work together.

THREE PHASES OF EROTIC RECOVERY

After an affair, your well-meaning family and friends may tell you things like, "once a cheater, always a cheater" or, "how can you ever trust them again?" They may encourage you to leave your partner. However, try not to make any major choices about your marriage or committed partnership right away.

In the early stages after the discovery of an affair, most people are in the Crisis Phase I, and there are two more phases to go through before you need to make any long-term decisions.

As long as you and your children are safe, treat yourself as if you have just been through a car wreck; you are probably feeling like your life has just been smashed to pieces. This time of upheaval will pass, if you get help and practice the skills you learn in each phase of recovery.

During the Crisis Phase I you will feel emotionally unstable, you may lose sleep, and might need to remind yourself to eat healthy and take care of yourself. You may have intrusive thoughts about the affair and demand to know details about your partner's infidelity.

This may lead to conflicts and even arguments. And yet, against your better judgment, you might be having more sex with one another than ever before; passionate and intense sex. You could be embarrassed to tell your therapist or your friends.

And you don't want your partner to think that this means they are forgiven.

Sex with your spouse or committed partner is normal after an affair and happens when you are both scared to lose one another. You may desperately want to connect, or want to hold each other. You may each crave the feeling of being intimate and in each other's arms.

Also, now that distance has been created between the two of you, you may find you are drawn to one another to use sex not only as comfort, but to express what is known in the animal kingdom as primal "Mate Guarding." It is a way to lay claim to one another when your monogamy has been threatened.

Although this can feel confusing, it is a natural result of a new relationship being formed – who is this person that you thought you knew? What was their outside affair partner attracted to that perhaps you hadn't seen in them?

You thought you knew everything about your partner, but now they are almost a stranger in some ways.

This feeling, although painful, can bring back a new sense of allure, a new longing and a sexual attraction that is emotionally loaded for both of you.

For others, there is no allure, and no sexual connection. During the Crisis Phase I, you may find there is so much betrayal, anger and resentment you can't imagine ever connecting to your partner again. Talk to your partner directly about your feelings.

Share with them if you don't feel ready to have sex. Maybe you are okay with some intimate physical time together, like holding each other in bed. Be honest. It is important to take your time and find other ways to feel safe as you move through the phases of recovery.

After your partner cheats, it may take time to recover your own self-esteem. One way to do this is to slow down the process and be assured that there is no pressure to have sex before you are ready. Whether you are sexual or shut off, this phase will pass.

You will recognize when you are entering phase two, the Insight Phase II, when you start referring to the infidelity as "our affair" instead of "your affair." There will be less blame and more curiosity. You will ask, "How did this happen to us?"

There will be less focus on the details of the affair, ("how many times did you meet with him, where did you have sex, were her boobs bigger than mine?") and you will focus on the emotional content of the affair ("were you thinking of me when you were with her/him?").

This is the time when couples therapy is invaluable. An expert in infidelity treatment can help you discern the reasons that the affair may have occurred in the first place.

In the Insight Phase II, the focus is on understanding each other and creating empathy. Don't try and find forgiveness right now.

That can be fleeting and temporary.

The one who has been cheated on will likely take back their forgiveness when they are feeling powerless, or when they need to rebalance the relationship.

Empathy is more important during this phase, and here you can begin to explore what real intimacy will look like going forward. Empathy means that both of you validate each other's feelings and begin to understand what it has been like to live in your worlds.

When you can experience empathy, you can begin to explore real erotic recovery. Eroticism becomes a new way to connect intimately and consciously. When that happens, the memory of the third person will no longer be in bed with you. In order to do this, you will begin to create a new sex life together, with new fantasies and new ways of being together.

You may begin to feel hopeful that your relationship can start over, and you can be together, in a better way. Some couples even say that the affair woke them up, and now they are closer than ever.

Phase III (three) is the Vision Phase of your recovery. Now is the time to decide if you want to create a new future for your relationship. You must both create a new monogamy agreement together. You will have to decide and negotiate what that new monogamy will look like.

This will include a new erotic life, one that is satisfying to both of you. This understanding is crucial to an exciting and passionate relationship.

If you ignore the erotic part of your relationship and focus only on getting along and avoiding conflict, you will find that you are good roommates, but you won't feel "in love" with your partner. Eventually you will feel dissatisfied and frustrated. It is through the erotic connection that you will each find that "in love" feeling.

But erotic connection takes work. Erotic recovery is a practice, like yoga or meditation. You have to practice it together and commit to a future of erotic recovery, every day.

BUILD INTIMACY
If you have decided that you want to have more sex, consider putting sex on your schedule. It may sound unromantic, but it can also be exciting and special if done the right way.

Scheduling gives you something to look forward to and shows a commitment to one another and your physical relationship.

Beyond sex, it's also important to explore other ways to build closeness that is often lost in low-sex or no-sex relationships. Physical intimacy doesn't only involve sex. Make an effort to renew your love and create that special spark.

Being close, both emotionally and physically, is an important part of a healthy relationship. And it's important to note that physical intimacy isn't limited to sex.

Spending more time together, whether you're curled up on the couch watching television or taking turns giving each other a massage, builds foundational intimacy. Here are other intimacy-building activities you might consider:

- Try a new activity together.
- Do something physical together such as going on a walk.
- Schedule on a vacation or getaway.
- Plan a staycation at home.
- Go on a scheduled date night.

GET HELP
Depending on the underlying causes, seeking outside help may also be a good option. You might try a marriage retreat, workshop, or seminar to help with communication and connection.

Consult a doctor to address any underlying medical conditions that may be impacting your sex life.

Seek support from a mental health professional together or separately to foster communication skills or learn stress management techniques.

If therapy feels like the right direction for you, consider seeing a counselor who focuses on sexual issues in marriage like a certified sex therapist. Your therapist can work with you to address any issues that are standing in the way of intimacy. Take these opportunities to focus on building a stronger, deeper marriage.

THE BENEFITS OF SEX

When you're having sex, you're unwittingly reaping the benefits of your sexual response cycle. Even though you're probably not thinking things like, "Wow, thank you, increased blood flow, for enabling more blood to rush to my vagina, resulting in mind-blowing sensations," that kind of process is part of what happens during sex to make it feel really good for you. (If sex doesn't feel good for you, you should read about painful sex to try to understand what's going on.)

Basically, when you're turned on or having sex, your body and brain are lighting up like a pinball machine, going through a multitude of physiologic changes to make sex as enjoyable as possible. This process is known as the sexual response cycle.

Experts usually categorize the sexual response cycle in four phases spanning from the second you get turned on (mentally or physically) to the blissful, tapped-out close of events. Different bodies of thought proceed through the sexual response cycle in slightly different ways, with some separating certain parts of the sexual response cycle that others lump together. Generally, though, here's what happens during sex to make it feel so damn good:

I. Desire (You start to really want sex.)

The feeling that you want to have sex, as the official start of the sexual response cycle, and for seriously good reason: It can be a huge part of getting mentally and physically ready for sex for some people. But it's also a pretty big area of sexual science interest because of how differently it can present in men and people with penises vs. women and people with vaginas.

"In the beginning of a relationship, many women do experience spontaneous desire the way it's portrayed in the media, as couples ripping each other's clothes off after a single sexy glance. "But research has borne out that for many women, desire is responsive, meaning that it responds to something that comes before it, [like physical arousal]."

So, for some people with vaginas (especially when in a shiny new relationship or when getting together with a new, exciting partner), desire might set off a sexual domino effect. But for others, desire may not kick in until after the sexual stuff has commenced (consensually, of course). Even though that may not go along with the typical portrayals of desire and sex, it's totally normal.

Here's what can happen if you experience desire as the first part of your sexual response cycle. Not every person will experience all of these during the desire, but it's a good general overview of the possibilities:

1. Your heart rate speeds up.

2. So does your breathing.

3. You might start to notice your skin flushing in areas like your chest and back. (This is fittingly called a "sex flush.)

4. "Your body releases more nitric oxide," This triggers effects like increasing blood supply to various parts of your body, including your vagina and cervix, he explains, which in turn leads to a multitude of other changes.

5. First up: the phenomenon sometimes called tenting, which is when your vagina dilates. The purpose of that dilation is theoretically to make it easier for a penis to fit in there, which

is unsurprisingly heteronormative, given human biology's purpose to continue the species.

The good thing is that even if you're having sex with someone who doesn't have a penis, this can make it easier for things like fingers and sex toys to fit inside you, too. There's also a theory that "[tenting] creates a sort of suctioning action that helps direct sperm to the cervix.

6. Made of the same kind of erectile tissue as a penis, your clitoris has the ability to get "erect" once it begins receiving that extra blood flow. This can make it more sensitive to stimulation.

7. Your labia minora (inner vaginal lips) also swell with extra blood.

8. As do your vaginal walls. (Sensing a pattern here?)

9. That extra blood flow also helps to increase vaginal lubrication, which can make insertion happen more easily and feel better to boot.

10. Also due to that excess blood flow, your nipples may become erect and feel more sensitive. In fact, all areas of your breasts might feel more sensitive the more turned on you get, so encourage your partner to explore. "Some things that may feel uncomfortable at [the] beginning of sex, like, oh, that itches, tickles, or hurts, may actually feel really good [as you get more turned on]."

11. Your muscles start tensing up in the buildup to eventual orgasm and the resulting physical release.

II. Arousal (Sexual stimulation starts to feel even better.)

This is sometimes known as the plateau phase, which isn't as boring as it sounds, we promise. Everything that was already happening before generally keeps happening, and a few new developments join in on the fun.

12. There's increased neurological activity in certain parts of the brain that are connected with sexual enjoyment. Although this is a research area that could benefit from some more scientific exploration, it appears as though parts of your brain like the amygdala (which helps you process emotions) may be involved.

13. This is often the phase where you get swept up enough that everyday stressors are fading into the background, which is often a key part of making way for orgasm, says Bill.

14. Your vagina is undergoing some seriously incredible changes, like your vaginal walls turning a deep purple color. That's probably hard to see (and stopping just to check it out might not be on your agenda), but the simple fact that it's happening is pretty cool.

15. Your muscles tense up even more....

16. Those muscle contractions might lead to straight-up spasms in body parts like your hands, feet, and face.

17. Your clitoris is becoming even more sensitive than it was before. Knowing what's good for it, it retracts under your clitoral hood to avoid becoming overstimulated.

II. Orgasm (You come. Or you don't. It's all good.)

Of course, sex can still be great even if you don't orgasm. Sometimes it can be frustrating if you don't orgasm. Sometimes it can even be both. If you do climax, everything basically goes off the rails physiologically in the best way possible.

18. Your heart rate, breathing, and blood pressure hit the ceiling. Each one peaks in a way it doesn't at any other point during sex.

19. "There's a big increase in the production of oxytocin. Oxytocin is a neurotransmitter related to, no surprise, increased feelings of pleasure and bonding.

20. Your muscles are convulsing hard. From your uterus to your vagina to your feet, muscles across your body are really going all out when it comes to those spasms.

21. Depending on how your body works, you might squirt, although when it occurs, it doesn't always happen in conjunction with orgasm.

22. A sudden, intense release of tension is a major orgasm characteristic, but it's worth noting that orgasms can feel different for different people (and even for the same people in different sexual experiences). Sometimes that release might be so strong you nearly black out, other times it might be a gentler whoosh—it just depends.

III. Resolution (You snuggle, fall asleep, or go again.)

23. It's pretty simple, really: With some time, basically everything from your heart rate to your breasts to your labia goes back to its usual color, size, and state.

While this resolution phase usually leads to a refractory period for people with penises (as in, a time when they physically can't have sex), that's not necessarily so for people with vaginas.

GOD MADE US MALE AND FEMALE

Let's start with Genesis 1:27-28:

So, God created man in His own image, in the image of God, He created him; male and female He created them. And God blessed them. And God said to them, "Be fruitful and multiply and fill the earth and subdue it, and have dominion over the fish of the sea and the birds of the heavens and over every living thing that moves on the earth."

In the act of creating "man in His own image" as male and female, God created human sexuality. It's His design. It's His idea, His gift to us. Our sexuality is connected to the fact that we are the same species but different in gender.

What does the Bible say about sex? The very first instruction God gives to the man and the woman in Genesis 1 is, "Be fruitful and multiply."

This command involves sexual engagement, on our part. God could have chosen another way to populate the earth, but He chose to make the sexual union part of His design, and He blessed that relationship.

We have to acknowledge there are cases where a married couple is unable to conceive. But infertility does not invalidate God's design.

So, the Lord God caused a deep sleep to fall upon the man, and while he slept took one of his ribs and closed up its place with flesh. And the rib that the Lord God had taken from the man He made into a woman and brought her to the man.

The man said, "This at last is bone of my bones and flesh of my flesh. She shall be called Woman, because she was taken out of Man."

Therefore, a man shall leave his father and his mother and hold fast to his wife, and they shall become one flesh.
(Genesis 2:21-24)

What I want you to see in this passage is that when God fashioned the woman to be a complement to the man, He was not yet done with the crescendo of His creation.

It's not until He brings the man and the woman back together again and "the two become one flesh" that we arrive at the summit. In that act of marriage and sexuality we see the pinnacle of creation.

I think there's something central and profound in the sexual act, as a part of a marriage designed by God. When a husband and wife become one flesh they experience a deep physical, emotional, and even spiritual oneness that binds them together.

But it does more than that. It also points to and reflects the goodness of God.

What does the Bible say about sex? The Bible makes it clear that this sexual bond is meant to happen within marriage. This, of course, is one point where our culture teaches a far different philosophy than God's Word.

Here are five reasons why a sexual relationship should occur within the confines of marriage:

1. Sex is meant to strengthen the marriage bond. In marriage, we enter into a covenant relationship with one another. This

covenant mirrors God's covenant. During the wedding ceremony, we vow to remain committed "for better or for worse, in sickness and in health, for richer or poorer ... till death do us part." These promises echo the promise God makes to us when He adopts us into His family and unites Himself to us in Christ. He has said that He will never leave us or forsake us.

God wants the husband and wife to be one. The recurring, ongoing participation in sex is the instrument that God uses so that we can experience a closer, richer, deeper relationship with one another.

When sex happens outside of the safe haven of a committed, loving covenant relationship—what used to be called "the bonds of matrimony" —you may still experience physical pleasure, but there will be an emptiness in your soul. There is something missing.

There is a shallowness to the sexuality that we experience apart from a lifelong covenant.

2. God wants to teach us more about the relationship between the Father, the Son, and the Spirit in the Trinity. There is oneness within the Trinity—there are three persons, but they are one. In marriage, there are two persons, but they become one.

In marriage, we learn something about the intimacy God enjoys within the context of the Trinity—the intimacy that the Father has with the Son, and the Son with the Spirit, and the Spirit with the Father and the Son.

3. God also wants to give us a picture of Christ's relationship with the Church. (Ephesians 5:22-33). In some mysterious way, the husband and wife relationship—and our sexuality—is tied to that picture.

4. A sexual relationship in marriage teaches us something about the nature of real love—God's love. Over a lifetime in marriage, we learn that in order for our sexuality to be expressed in the way that God intends it, the sexuality needs to be unselfish.

Both husband and wife must be committed to pleasing each other and meeting each other's needs.

5. It is best for the offspring of our sexual union to grow up in a home governed by a covenant relationship between a husband and a wife who love one another and are committed to each other. If a child is growing up in a setting where there is one parent or where two parents are not bound together in covenant love with one another, that child is missing something.

Consider this: If our sexual relationship is this powerful and this important, is it any wonder that Satan would take delight in trying to undermine, pervert, and destroy our human sexuality?

Is it any wonder that sex is so huge, so pervasive in our culture—and that the temptation to operate independently of God's plan is so powerful?

NOT HAVING SEX LEAD TO DIVORCE?

While there is a lack of recent research on the topic, older studies have shown that lower sexual satisfaction and sexual frequency are associated with marriages breaking up.

According to a 2015 study published in Social Psychological and Personality Science, having more sex indicates greater well-being for people in relationships, but only up to once a week. In the study, more than that did not.

Being dissatisfied with your sex life can breed trouble for a relationship. That is to say that the lack of sex itself isn't necessarily an issue, but rather any dissatisfaction associated with the lack of sex is.

If you're unsatisfied with the amount of sex you and your partner are having, you may be wondering whether your relationship can be sustained. Making the decision to end your marriage can be very complex.

There are many different factors that can contribute to feeling sexually satisfied in a partnership, and they can differ from person to person.

RELATIONSHIP CHANGES AFTER INFIDELITY

You can't trust anything anymore

Not surprisingly, not only will a victim of infidelity mistrust their partner sexually and emotionally, he or she might also begin to doubt them in other areas.

"In the wake of an affair, more and more lies come out, and that makes trust very difficult. "It then becomes easy to feel dubious toward your partner in other aspects of life, such as finances or parenting."

Your confidence plummets—or soars

Cheating can create a level of stress and anxiety that can trigger a depressive episode. "For some people, an affair can make them lose focus on other aspects of their life. Self-care, their career trajectory, friendships, and thoughtful parenting can all take a backseat." "Take it one day at a time and start prioritizing healthy habits, like going to the gym and starting therapy, to help you rebuild your life and your relationship."

On the other hand, the wake of an affair can actually help you focus on yourself.

"People who recover from infidelity are usually able to go within themselves and recapture their center of power." "They actually end up stronger and more resilient than before the affair." One Atlanta, GA man who discovered his wife was cheating feels like he finally found himself once his unhappy marriage came to an end.

"For the first time in years I was able to dedicate time to myself—going the gym, wearing better clothes, focusing on my health and simply because I wasn't depressed that I was stuck in a terrible marriage anymore," he says. "I finally had the energy to start fixing myself instead of devoting my efforts to fixing my marriage." (Your brain isn't immune to a rocky relationship. See how your brain reacts to the ups and downs of love, exclusively on Prevention Premium.)

You may not even recognize your libido

For some people, infidelity can destroy their sex life. "If your partner has cheated on you, even if you are working hard to forgive and rebuild the relationship, sex is often the last piece of the puzzle." "You're sorting through all kinds of emotions— depression, anger, betrayal—and that just kills your sexual desire."

But an affair can also bolster your libido—even if you're not the one doing the cheating. One father of two from Atlanta found that he was more attracted to his wife than ever when he discovered she was having an affair.

"It was almost as if I felt in competition for my wife's affections and I had to win her back from him," he says.

"We had a lot of wild sex, often following explosive arguments about the affair," he says. And that's not surprising. "Sex can be a powerful way to heal after cheating." "It helps make an insecure relationship feel temporarily safe and intimate."

Or perhaps after living in a relatively unhappy relationship your sexual appetite will be boosted simply by the excitement of being with a new, more attentive partner. "Because my wife and I had been together so long, and from such a young age, I didn't realize that I was actually attractive to other women and that I could be attracted to them, too," says one man from New York

New York. For him, dating and sex with new partners after his wife's affair boosted his sex drive.

"Part of the reason many people cheat is because they felt unwanted or unloved in their relationship. Then they discover sexual or emotional appreciation in the affair which, in turn, bolsters their confidence."

The flip side: The person who is being cheated on will suffer a major blow to his or her self-esteem, points out Rod.

"After being cheated on by my Wife, at first I felt embarrassed and like I just wasn't enough. Not attractive, smart, or funny enough," says a father of two from College Park. (We asked a private investigator and here are 8 signs of a cheater)

The unexpectedly good news is that those feelings of inadequacy didn't last long—at least for him. He and his wife spent some time apart and once he started dating again, he was reminded that he was lovable and desirable.

"Oddly, getting cheated on completely changed my self-confidence for the better, and I've been able to hang onto that feeling ever since," he says.

In fact, he points to his renewed sense of self-confidence as one of the reasons he was able to eventually reconcile with his wife.

Your focus totally shifts.

SEX ISN'T WORKING FOR ME

Whether being in a sexless partnership is a deal breaker depends on the couple. But if you find yourself in a sexless marriage or you're dissatisfied with the amount of sex you and your partner are having, the first step is to communicate that with your partner and explore ways that you can find the intimacy that each of you needs to feel fulfilled.

There are many reasons that a relationship can become sexless, and many are treatable. Experiencing sexual issues in a relationship can be very difficult, but you don't have to manage it alone.

What is sexual dysfunction?

- When you have problems with sex, doctors call it "sexual dysfunction." Men and women can have it. There are four kinds of sexual problems in women.

- Desire disorders. If you have a desire disorder you may not be interested in having sex. Or, you may have less desire for sex than you used to.

- Arousal disorders. When you don't feel a sexual response in your body or you start to respond but can't keep it up, you might have an arousal disorder.

- Orgasmic disorders. If you can't have an orgasm or you have pain during orgasm, you may have an orgasmic disorder.

- Sex pain disorders. When you have pain during or after sex, you may have a sex pain disorder. In some women, the muscles in the outer part of the vagina tighten when you start to have sex. A man's penis or a vibrator can't get into the tight vagina.

What causes sexual dysfunction?

- Medicines, diseases (like diabetes or high blood pressure), alcohol use, or vaginal infections can cause sexual problems.
- Depression, an unhappy relationship or abuse (now or in the past) can also cause sexual problems.
- You may have less sexual desire during pregnancy, right after childbirth or when you are breast-feeding. After menopause, many women feel less sexual desire, have vaginal dryness or have pain during sex.
- The stresses of everyday life can affect your ability to have sex. Being tired from a busy job or caring for young children may make you feel less desire to have sex. Or, you may be bored by a long-standing sexual routine.

How do I know if I have a problem?

Up to 70 percent of couples have a problem with sex at some time. Most women sometimes have sex that doesn't feel good. This doesn't mean you have a sexual problem.

If you don't want to have sex or it never feels good, you might have a sexual problem. The best person to decide if you have a sexual problem is you! Discuss your worries with your doctor. Remember that anything you tell your doctor is private.

What can I do?

To improve your desire, change your usual routine. You may want to rent an erotic video or read a "sexy" book with your partner.

Arousal disorders can be helped if you use a vaginal cream for dryness. Mineral oil also works. If you have gone through menopause, talk to your doctor about taking estrogen.

If you have a problem having an orgasm, masturbation can help you. Extra stimulation (before you have sex with your partner) with a vibrator may be helpful.

You might need rubbing or stimulation for up to an hour before having sex. Many women don't have an orgasm during intercourse. If you want an orgasm with intercourse, you or your partner may want to gently stroke your clitoris.

If you're having pain during sex, try different positions. When you are on top, you have more control over penetration and movement. Empty your bladder before you have sex. Try using extra creams or try taking a warm bath before sex. If your sex pain doesn't go away, talk to your doctor.

If you have a tight vagina, you can try using something like a tampon to help you get used to relaxing your vagina. Your doctor can tell you more about this.

What else can I do?

Learn more about your body and how it works. Ask your doctor about how medicines, illnesses, surgery, age, pregnancy or menopause can affect sex.

Practice "sensate focus" exercises where one partner gives a massage, while the other partner says what feels good and requests changes (example: "lighter," "faster," etc).

Fantasizing may increase your desire. Squeezing the muscles of your vagina tightly and then relaxing them may increase your arousal.

Try sexual activity other than intercourse, such as massage, oral sex or masturbation.

What about my partner?

Talk with your partner about what each of you like and dislike, or what you might want to try. Ask for your partner's help. Remember that your partner may not want to do some things you want to try. Or, you may not want to try what your partner wants.

You should respect each other's comforts and discomforts.

This helps you and your partner have a good sexual relationship. If you can't talk to your partner, your doctor or a counselor may be able to help you.

If you feel like a partner is abusing you, you should tell your doctor.

How can my doctor help?

Talk to your doctor about your sexual health. Explain your problems openly and honestly. Your doctor can also give you ideas about treating your sexual problems or can refer you to a sex therapist or counselor if it is needed.

How Long Is Too Long without Sex in a Relationship?

If you're in a romantic relationship, chances are sex plays an important role. It's an intimate way of connecting that

91

relationship experts say can often be the glue that holds two people together for the long haul. However, it's quite common for sex to change over the course of a long-term relationship—both in terms of quality and frequency.

Relationship researchers and therapists call the early stage of a new relationship the "LIMERENCE" or "honeymoon" stage, which lasts anywhere from three months to two years. This is the stage that most couples thrive in—and this is true of men and women as well as non-binary individuals.

"Hollywood knows this, and capitalizes on our longing, which is why many movies focus on the dramatic tension bringing couples together, but few showcases those sometimes-awkward evenings when one partner tries to initiate sex and the other turns them down." "During this stage, we're flooded with hormones, chemicals and newfound excitement that leads very easily to sex (and lots of it)."

However, that, at this early stage of a relationship, the couple often does not know each other all too well, which means each is on their best behavior and showcasing their positive qualities.

"This makes it very easy to center our fantasies about the other person and the relationship in our view, so some of what we're having sex with isn't the actual person in front of us, but a romanticized, fantasy version of them and what this relationship might become."

"As we spend more time with someone, the early relationship hormones fade and real life starts to set in, so start to see the other person's humanness and all of their imperfections."

It's also true that, as a relationship develops and time passes, other areas of life start to take greater priority, such as school, work, and family obligations, which is another reason why many couples don't make it past the Limerence stage.

During this stage's end, a couple is often having less sex than they were before. "Some are destined to fail from the beginning, but others could have made it last if they understood this occurs in every relationship and how to deepen their connection."

One great way to keep the spark alive is by having sex—lots of it. "Sex is form of connection and bonding in addition to obviously providing us with (hopefully) a lot of physical and emotional pleasure that's good for mind, body, and soul."

"During sex, we release a hormone called oxytocin, that has been nicknamed the 'love hormone' because it facilitates pair bonding among couples."

HOW MUCH SEX WE NEED AND HOW LONG?

The good news for most non-married or married couples reading this book is that experts say there's really no one ideal sexual frequency; no one amount of sex that works for everyone. One couple may find that enough sex is simply one to two times a week, while another might find that enough sex is one to two times a month. In fact, it really depends on the couples, their preferences, and their life pressures.

Research published in the journal Archives of Sexual Behavior found that the average couple has sex about 54 times a year, which comes out to about once a week. And another study published in the journal Social Psychological and Personality Science found that once a week was the gold standard for relationship happiness.

"Regularity of sex becomes a situation where couples can collaborate instead of compromise," with Manhattan Wellness. "If one partner feels satisfied with having sex daily and the other feels satisfied having sex once a week, how they unite to to find joy in intimacy, potentially expanding their ideas and discussions around sex, can lead to both members of the couple gaining a sense of satisfaction and a grow the intimate connection."

Simply cohabiting without sex is not enough. "If two healthy people are in a relationship, live together, and yet do not have sex, they sound more like roommates than lovers, points out."

"'It's just sex, and there is so much more to a marriage than sex,' some might argue, but a couple's sexual intimacy is a reflection of the relationship."

There are a few stipulations, however, one of them being the postpartum period, or the one-year period after a woman has a baby. During the postpartum period, there is often a lack of intimacy in terms of sex. "With postpartum intimacy in relationships sex, in terms of vaginal penetration, requires medical clearance which depending on the birth of the child could range from a few weeks to several months to allow optimal healing."

"That being said, after children hormonally the female sex drive naturally shifts, this could account for an increase or decrease in sexual desire."

Life transitions can also have a massive part in sex drive, as well as each partner's sexual needs. "If one partner is feeling increased stress or anxiety, or feeling insecure within other realms of their life such as a job or financial concerns, this can hinder someone's sexual drive or ability to connect intimately with their partner."

"During these times, sexual activity can slow down, if not stall altogether, and last the entire span of the stressful period of time."

AFTER THE AFFAIR

Resuming physical intimacy after an affair is one of the most intensely emotionally loaded of all human experiences. I'm defining the word "affair" as extramarital sexual relations, or sexual relations outside of a relationship between partners who have lived together for at least one year. (In the context of a dating relationship, I would label this situation "cheating".)

Thinking about resuming sexual relations after the revelation of an affair can fill a partner with anticipation and longing, or mixed feelings, even dread. The post-affair experience is, for both partners, but especially for the one receiving the news (the Receiver), a time of simultaneous challenges to live as a high-functioning adult Self, close on the heels of what amounts to a small trauma.

There is no "right" or "wrong" way to resume Intimacy after an affair, just as there are no right or wrong answers to the many questions and dilemmas a couple must face after the revelation of an affair. There's guaranteed not to be enough time to process all of the thoughts and feelings, questions and dilemmas at a time like this.

The decision whether and when to resume involves some conscious thinking and some purposeful steps, but is probably also going to be based on gut reactions and listening to your intuition. The following ideas are offered to assist couples on their way to restoring their intimacy as a couple, but just as importantly, to help each of them to restore their own personal sexual wholeness.

The decision whether or not to resume sexual intimacy after an affair is not a foregone conclusion, and neither partner should ever be pressured to resume sex before they know that their body is ready, feel that they want to resume, and feel that it is the right thing to do. The decision involves the body, the heart, and one's sense of fairness and justice.

One of the most critical experiences for both partners is to receive and accept empathy for their current experience, preferably from a neutral party such as a psychotherapist. It may be surprising that both partners need empathy after the revelation of an affair, not just the Receiver. But both partners are going through an emotional upheaval at this time, and both need acknowledgment of what they are going through.

First, let's consider the body. If the affair was brief or just started recently, then it is quite likely that the other partner finds out about it by having symptoms of an STD, which are then confirmed by a physician.

Even more traumatic, but just as commonly, there were no symptoms, but one partner finds out from a routine blood test at a doctor's office, that he or she has an STD. Any STD's must be treated before sexual relations can resume.

It's also a really good idea to meet with a psychotherapist to process your reactions at this time. Beyond this, all other recommendations should be implemented as soon as possible, but wouldn't need to happen before resuming sex.

It's a good idea for both partners to understand how their body reacts to stress, and take care of their body accordingly. Stress-related health problems such as reduced immunities, slip-and-fall accidents, ulcers, tension headaches and migraines, and intestinal problems can all flare up at this time.

Good self-care is crucial, including adequate rest, good nutrition, the right form exercise, sunlight, and the appropriate medications. It may be tempting to talk late into the night trying to resolve the issues, for example, but your rest is much more important.

Sexual problems, such as lack of desire, arousal, or ability to climax should be verbally acknowledged, and both partners should be prepared to make healthy accommodations to the other's needs. The body can feel numb at this time, and the senses dulled and slowed down. This is often a sign of trauma, can be felt by either or both partners, and usually goes away on its own, after a few months.

NEXT IS THE HEART AND SOUL
Both partners might be brokenhearted. For the one who had the affair, there might be heartbreak about the damage done to the marriage; but there might also be heartbreak about losing the affair, or having to choose between the spouse and the lover. There are significant feelings of rejection for both partners.

The receiver can feel the deepest isolating rejection a human being can ever feel. That although they have given themselves to the other exclusively, and although they were available to their partner, their partner went outside the marriage for sex. The one involved in the affair often finds that the affair ends abruptly when it is exposed, and they are feeling that loss.

They might soon lose their marriage too.

The void that the affair filled suddenly becomes a gaping void once again. It can be very healing to be accepted once again by the receiving partner, if he or she is ready; but that can take time. Both partners can vacillate between intense desire to win back their spouse, to intense desire to be free from the spouse. Finally, both partners begin to think about the fairness and justice of resuming sex.

Is it right to resume, and under what conditions?

Should the involved one apologize, and is that enough?

It is normal to momentarily desire humiliation for our partner, or even to daydream about it. But in real life, is that ever good, or right?

Does it help either of you to heal?

Should the receiving partner apologize for anything they might have done to cause the involved partner to be vulnerable to getting involved in the affair?

How do the religious beliefs of both parties come into play here?

It takes most people about a year of hard work to sort out the issues of their body, heart, and fairness after the revelation of an affair. While they are on their healing journey, if the couple decides to resume ongoing sexual relations, the experience is going to have a slightly different meaning for each of them, each time they are together.

It may be stating the obvious, but couples find it quite difficult to communicate verbally at this time, without stalemates, silences, and shouting.

Resuming sexual relations can provide another means of communication. Sometimes the body can express what words cannot.

Sexual intimacy after an affair can help to answer one of the biggest questions after an affair, "Should I stay or should I go?"

It can provide the most supreme comfort, or it can leave either partner feeling very alone. The sexual bond is, in the end, how couples give life to the next generation. Love and commitment, symbolized in the sexual act, energize the couple, empowering them to give beyond themselves.

This principle holds true for all healthy committed couples — birth parents and adoptive parents, heterosexual or same-sex couples, and non-parent couples.

Once both partners have had the opportunity to receive empathy, to feel heard and understood in their experience, then they can learn to turn towards each other again and speak genuinely and authentically to each other.

I encourage my clients to use Heart Statements when they get to this point in recovering from an affair.

A Heart Statement is a verbalization to your partner, about what's going on inside of you emotionally. When you tell your partner how you're feeling right now, or how you're affected by a situation, this allows your partner to hear you on a deep heart level.

Working Towards Intimacy

Most couples understand intuitively that if they are going to try to rebuild their marriage after an affair, then healthy, positive and exclusive sexual intimacy is the foundation for moving forward together. Once they have both had the opportunity to begin addressing some of the issues of the body, heart, and meaning, they usually both feel the need to resume sexual relations. Most significantly, it is an attempt at starting over, starting fresh.

At times the sexual connection can signal ownership, especially in the mind of the one who did not have an affair. At times it can signal contrition, a desire for forgiveness; or it can be a gesture of forgiveness. Both might be carrying some things that they want forgiveness for, and some things they wish to offer forgiveness for.

In other words, if the healing process progresses well, there begins to be less of a clear dualism, less labeling of a "good guy" and "bad guy".

There is less emphasis on feeling punished, or feeling victimized. There is more of a real-life acceptance that people are not all good, or all bad, and they both gain deeper maturity by working through this healing process.

The receiving and giving of EMPATHY plays a huge role in getting to this point. When both partners make a good faith effort, in the bedroom and outside of it, to listen attentively and use heart statements, they get to know each other's heart better, and begin to reestablish oneness.

I mentioned that most couples feel the need to resume sexual relations, once they have acknowledged the areas of body, heart and meaning. But what about the desire to resume, the ability to feel aroused, and the ability to climax?

Desire is all about feeling prioritized. There is no amount of gift-giving, wining and dining, and being a good and responsible partner that can take the place of simply looking into your partner's eyes again, and letting your shared gaze tell them that they are first in your heart.

In fact, when partners give lavish gifts, start working out again, or make big promises, the other partner tends to see it as a temporary form of manipulation. The oneness is lost, and desire plummets. If you can't look into your partner's eyes, or allow them to look into yours, then self-check for the reasons why.

Perhaps shame or anger, or some other difficult emotion, is still holding you back. Talk to your partner about your feelings, and listen well when they talk about their feelings.

Once you are able to re-establish gaze, then add the element of touch.

Hugging and/or kissing at the five key points of the day — upon waking, leaving the home for the day's work, returning home in the evening, evening meal, and bedtime— allows you to re-discover your chemical attraction to each other.

Once chemical attraction is re-established for both partners, then it becomes much easier to enjoy the other person for who they are, participate in your shared interests, and feel more compatible. The marriage begins to feel exclusive again.

There is less desire for outside help from friends, family and a therapist, and more desire for time alone together, and desire resurfaces. This sets the stage for teamwork in helping each other through any problems with arousal.

For a man, erectile dysfunction can be a problem at this time, due to mixed feelings and being unsure about the future of the marriage. There are lots of non-prescription ways to work through this problem.

These include the "Squeeze Technique", acceptance of variations in size of the erection during the course of lovemaking, and lengthening the duration of lovemaking, the "Penis as a Paintbrush Technique" and many more.

Women who have had arousal problems report that talking about it in the moment helps, as well as having all distractions removed, such as chores, child and elder care, and work responsibilities.

Side note: ALL couples need to start thinking of sex as an airplane taking off or landing, which means you must turn off all electronic devices!

Climax can still be an issue, and although it may sound counterintuitive, climax starts with setting the scene for lovemaking. Rebuilding couples need a private retreat with no reminders of the third person. New sheets are a must, especially if the third person was in the bed.

Rebuilding couples report that new paint, changing the furniture arrangement, and establishing a little ritual can all help.
A ritual might be something as simple as lighting two new white candles, to symbolize a fresh beginning, and the energy that comes from your love and commitment.

Reading a favorite poem or piece of wisdom literature aloud together can be part of the ritual too. It's also helpful to develop "our special touches", such as hand massage, foot massage, or a form of genital touch that you haven't tried before.

"Our special touches" make foreplay a way to communicate your love and commitment, and not just a warm-up exercise.

A word here about "toys" and fantasy play. Couples report that toys are enjoyable once in a while, but that with regular use, they can have a displacing effect, whereby one or both partners find that their body is more stimulated by the toy than by their spouse's touch. Most importantly for rebuilding couples, the toy can very easily represent a third entity in the bedroom, which is the last thing on earth they need at this time.

It can be very tempting for both partners to engage in fantasy play around the third person. Re-enacting the love triangle may seem as if it will help you process the trauma, make you more attractive to your spouse, or create titillation. But re-enacting the triangle consistently creates new hurts and reduces trust.

The most healing, trust, and satisfying sex comes from talking and acting as if you are the only two people in the world, from the time you set the stage, until after you have both climaxed and rested together.

When couples work together thoughtfully to re-establish their individual and joint sexual wholeness after an affair, they are then able to get back to telling their joint story, "The Story of Us". The energy shared and gained through their intimacy re-establishes their unity.

They renew their desire to not only voice support during each

other's ups and downs, successes and setbacks, joys and sorrows, but to be an integral part of all of these. With this new sense of shared meaning as their foundation, the couple's energy then can be shared in healthy ways with family, friends, co-workers and the community.

Of course, this is an optimistic rendering of sexual and emotional healing within the context of renewed commitment and a so-called happy ending.

SETBACKS AND HURTS

Couples who are rebuilding physical and emotional intimacy after an affair deserve a lot of respect for the courageous work they are doing each and every day, towards individual healing and healing the relationship. The Story of Us now has some very pain-filled chapters.

Setbacks and hurts can seem to undo all of the good that the couple is doing. The frustration, hurt and other painful, forceful emotions caused by setbacks and hurts can put one or both partners into a fight-or-flight response, or even create a stunned "deer in the headlights" reaction.

But individuals and marriages do have the ability to recover from follow-up setbacks. The following are some typical setbacks to healing after an affair. All of them can affect the desire, arousal and climax phases of emotional intimacy.

Going to couple's therapy, but your spouse refuses to go. The spouse who had the affair might refuse on the grounds that the therapist will take sides against him/her. Another reason can be that a partner is holding a secret about money, work, substances, or a lie that has been told.

The spouse who didn't have the affair might be feeling like a "loser", or "ugly", is worried that the therapist will want her to talk about what he/she might have done to contribute to the affair happening.

Refusing to go to couple's therapy could be about power and control, it could be about revenge, or it could be about not being in love any more. As important as couple's therapy is at a time like this, it is vastly more important to get to know your partner's heart better. Instead of issuing an ultimatum, try asking your partner how she/he felt inside when you suggested going to couple's therapy.

If they are willing to explain, then listen to their whole answer and thank them for being willing to talk about it. Go to therapy on your own, and invite your spouse to join you.

You and your spouse have warped perceptions

What is beautiful, such as your body, might seem ugly. What was joyful, such as being together sexually, now feels sad, or stressful. A marriage that was once full of exciting possibilities, now feels like a trap or a jail.

Warped perceptions are often the result of trauma. The trauma of learning about the affair, or the shock of being suddenly exposed in an affair, can even touch on childhood traumas. Remind yourself of ways that you have overcome shocks, adverse experiences and setbacks in the past, to remind yourself where your strengths lie.

When friends and allies affirm you, accept the affirmation.

You deserve to feel good again, even if you're the one who had the affair.

Dreaming about your spouse affair

You can't stop imagining your spouse and the intruder doing things together.

You imagine them sharing an elegant meal at a restaurant, having sex, or enjoying long intimate conversations.

The partner who had the affair may be thinking about the things they did together, but may try to hide in these thoughts. Both partners can feel very shut out. Reach out to your partner with touch or words when you think about the intruder.

You don't have to talk about the thoughts unless you want to; you can talk about any topic, or simply reach out with touch. It is healthy to process these thoughts with a therapist.

4. Forgiveness seems far, far away, even impossible

The hurt just seems too big to ever get past, and too much about your marriage has been damaged by the affair. The pressure to forgive quickly is a symptom of our high-speed post-modern age. We would like to microwave everything!

Forgiveness is a process, and can't be rushed. Use this time to get resourced on the subject of forgiveness.

Allow yourself to feel whatever you feel, without judgment.

Emotion Is a Teacher

Forgiveness accesses the spiritual part of a person, allowing you to regain a sense of personal meaning. Nurture your spiritual life at this time, by reading wisdom literature, engaging in prayer, meditation, and yoga, and by consulting with a spiritual mentor if you have one.

The healing of sexual intimacy is tied in with these setbacks, but in a different way for each couple, and each person. The body, heart and meaning all work together in the process of recovering from the affair.

SEX IS A BASIC HUMAN URGE

Neither men, nor women and survive without our basic human needs. They are food, liquids, sleep and such. We will die if we don't get these. Giving in to urges however are not necessary for survivals.

I might have an urge to pee while being on a busy street. But if I suppress this urge and wait until later, I will still survive. I might have an urge to call a person who claim all men are rapists and ignorant asshole, but I can survive just fine without saying anything.

I might see someone with a nice smartphone that I want, but I survive just fine without taking the phone.

It can be annoying not giving in to our urges, because urges are much about instincts and pleasure. But it is very possible and it is actually something we start learning around the age of 2, so I can't see why it would be difficult for a grown man.

No urge is irrepressible. People don't die without sex. We can control our actions.

About ejaculation. Expired sperm cells in the testicles need to be removed every now and then. The body ejaculating the expired cells, have nothing to do with sex. The body will often choose to do it during sleep when other clean up and healing processes are being done too. No sex needed.

(And men are not more honey than women. We just hide it better because we have been told our whole life that we are indecent sluts if we admit we want sex several times a day.)

OVERCOMING AVERSION TO SEX

The symptoms of aversion to sex are fear of engaging in sex, trying to make the sex act as short as possible, finding that you need to build up your confidence and resolve before sex just to get through it, thinking of excuses to avoid or postpone sex, and feeling ill just prior to sex and somewhat depressed afterward.

Some people actually experience panic attacks while engaged in sex. Your symptom of revulsion at the very thought of having sex is also a typical symptom.

Any of the symptoms of sexual aversion will interfere with your ability to meet your husband's need.

How can you meet his need for sex if you have even one of these reactions?

You can't. You must completely overcome the aversion if you ever hope to enjoy a sexual experience with your husband. And then be certain that the conditions that led to your aversion are never repeated.

Remember how you developed the aversion in the first place? You associated a certain behavior, having sex, with an unpleasant emotional reaction to something your husband did to you. Eventually the unpleasant reaction was triggered whenever you even thought about having sex with your husband, and certainly whenever you made love.

To overcome the aversion, you must break the association of sex with your husband from the unpleasant emotional reaction. The easiest way to do that is to associate sex with the state of relaxation.

Those without a sexual aversion may suggest that you take the direct route: Try to relax next time you make love. However, you and anyone else experiencing this hardship knows that the direct route is usually impossible to follow.

The very thought of having sex with your husband probably puts you in a state of near-panic.

So that's where we will begin — with your thoughts.

Step 1: Learn to relax when you think about sex.
The exercises that I am recommending to you will require about 15 minutes of your time every day. It is very important that you not miss a day, because the process will not work as well if you allow time gaps in the procedure.

Sit in a comfortable chair in a room by yourself with your eyes closed. If possible, play relaxing music in the background. Think of various experiences that you have had. Some of them will help you relax and others will make you feel tense. If you have an aversion to sex, whenever you think about making love, you will probably feel your tension rise and it will definitely feel unpleasant to you.

Stop thinking about sex, and redirect your thoughts to relaxing experiences. Then focus on relaxing each muscle in your body. Begin with your feet and move all the way up to your head, focusing your attention on relaxing every muscle along the way. It may take you five minutes or more before you know that all of your muscles are fully relaxed.

When you are completely relaxed, think about making love again, but this time remain completely relaxed. Don't allow any muscle to tense up. As you think about sex, you will notice that some thoughts don't bother you at all, but others, like making love to your husband, may make it almost impossible to remain relaxed.

Don't think about making love to your husband just yet. Think only about sex, in general. Leave your husband out of your thoughts altogether. Investigate your own reactions to sex by imagining various aspects of sex. If you have any sexual fantasies, think about them, and what it is that makes them appealing to you.

Then, without thinking of your husband, think about other aspects of sex that are less appealing or downright unappealing.

Be completely relaxed while you are thinking of all of these things. When your first fifteen minutes relaxation exercise is over, take notes of what you learned about yourself.

What sexual thoughts were appealing to you, and what thoughts were unappealing?

What thoughts made you feel relaxed, and what thoughts made it difficult for you to relax?

The contents of this journal should not be shared with your husband until your sexual aversion is completely overcome and you have a mutually fulfilling sexual relationship with him.

If there were certain sexual thoughts (not related to your husband) that made your muscles feel tense, or made your stomach feel tight, repeat this 15-minute exercise each day until you can think about them without feeling tense. You should also journal after each session to help you think through the reactions you are experiencing.

Step 2: Learn to relax when you think about having sex with your husband. If you have an aversion to sex with your husband, you will feel an unpleasant tension whenever you think of making love to him. So, in this step, the goal is to be able to think about it without feeling tension or experiencing an unpleasant reaction.

As I've already explained, an aversive reaction is created when an unpleasant emotional reaction is associated with a situation or behavior. The way to reverse that association is to try to stop the unpleasant reaction from occurring when the situation or behavior is present. If you can feel relaxed just thinking about sex with your spouse, that also tends to "extinguish" the aversive association that was previously made.

Close your eyes, sit back, and relax. Be certain you are alone and without anything or anyone to distract you. Relax all your muscles from head to toe as you did before, and think about making love with your husband.

You will notice that certain thoughts are more upsetting than others. It could be that one of the ways your husband wants to make love is particularly upsetting to you. (The thought of him forcing his hand over your body, particularly putting it between your legs raises your anxiety level.)

Eventually you will find that even thoughts of the most upsetting sex acts will no longer elicit an unpleasant reaction.

That's because with proper relaxation, you can extinguish your emotional reactions to almost anything.

The information you learn about yourself in this step will help you in the next step, so be sure to continue taking notes in your journal after each 15-minute session. You should document aspects of lovemaking with your husband that create the greatest stress for you.

Even though you will learn to be relaxed when you think about them, you will not want to repeat them when you get back to making love to him again.

Step 3: Learn to relax when you think about having sex with your husband with him in the same room. As soon as you have learned to be relaxed when thinking about making love to your husband, you are ready for the next step, inviting him to join you in the same room.

At first, he should simply sit somewhere else in the room and read a book. Even though he is not paying much attention to you, you may need to start practicing relaxation all over again. His very presence may make you tense.

If you relax all of your muscles from head to toe, you will eventually find yourself comfortable once again. Then, as you think about making love to him, continue to relax.

At this stage, your husband should not say or do anything but sit and read a book. If he cannot follow that simple instruction, we have serious problems. The reason you have a sexual aversion is that he has tried to make love to you in a way that is enjoyable for him, but unpleasant for you.

To overcome your sexual aversion, he will need to learn to take your feelings into account when he makes love to you in the future. But in this step, if he refuses to follow the assignment, and instead of quietly reading, he starts talking to you, or walks over and touches you, stop the procedure entirely. There is no hope for a successful transition to sex with your husband if he cannot follow your simplest requests.

It is essential for your husband to understand that you, not he, must be in complete control of your recovery process or it will not work. If he cannot or will not agree to that, it not only explains why you have the aversion to begin with, but also explains how his lack of cooperation has prevented your recovery.

Continue these exercises every day until you are completely relaxed thinking about making love to your husband with him in the same room. And don't forget to take notes in your journal that describe your experience.

Step 4: Learn to relax when you talk to your husband about having sex with him. Now you are ready to tell your husband what you are thinking. Sit back in your comfortable chair and close your eyes. At first, limit your description to sexual situations that you find easy to talk about, and avoid talking about those sex acts that you find particularly disturbing. When you first start talking about sex, you will find your tension rising again, but after a little practice, you will learn to be relaxed as you describe your feelings.

He should say nothing to you as you talk to him. All he should do is listen, if your husband decides to take charge, and tries to talk you into making love to him after you describe your thoughts, tell him that it is that very thing that created the aversion in the first place.

If he cannot follow the steps, end it.

Eventually, you should describe as many sexual situations to your husband as you can think of. You may want to refer to your journal to help you remember what some of them were. Whenever you talk about them, try to remain completely relaxed, and you will eventually find that even your most disturbing sexual memories will no longer elicit a tense or anxious response.

Step 5: Learn to relax when you make love to your husband. You should ease into a sexual relationship with your husband very slowly and comfortably. Continue to spend 15 minutes each day on this assignment so that you do not lose momentum.

First, you should learn to become comfortable with affection, being able to hug, kiss and hold hands without any fear that it will lead to sex. Then, have your husband rub your arms, feet and lower legs, backs, and other non-erogenous zones (avoid breast, stomach and genital areas), again without it leading to sex. Do the same for him.

When you are comfortable being touched by your husband in non-erogenous zones, and you are comfortable touching him, you are ready to begin the first stages of making love.

I have not discussed feelings of sexual arousal with you, because our goal was to overcome aversive reactions. But by the time you are able to talk to your husband about having sex with him while feeling completely relaxed you may have already started to experience feelings of sexual arousal.

The affection you experienced may also have led to feelings of sexual arousal. That feeling of sexual arousal is your signal to make love to your husband.

Don't ever try to make love without it.

Remember, if any aspect of lovemaking is unpleasant to you, figure out a way of making it enjoyable. Have your husband rub your back in a way that you enjoy, not just a way that he enjoys.

Resist the temptation to go ahead and make love just to make your husband happy, because it is likely to set you back.

Remember, if this is not successful, you will probably go back to not making love at all.

When you are ready for intercourse, have your husband lay entirely motionless on his back at first. Sit or lay on top of him so that you are in complete control of the situation. Experiment with different positions and methods of intercourse so that you can learn how your body works to create the most enjoyable feelings.

Only relinquish control to him after he has become educated in what it is that enables you to enjoy the experience with him.

Sometimes you will experience what behaviorists call "spontaneous recovery," because your habits will all be very new. Spontaneous recovery is when you suddenly feel the old aversive reactions without any warning. When that happens, it just means that there are residual effects still present that crop up from time to time.

You'll find that these unexpected intrusions will decrease over time until they hardly ever occur. Amazingly enough, if you understand how to turn lovemaking into an enjoyable experience, you will probably want to make love more often than your husband does. Why?

Because the more you enjoy something, the more you will want to do it. That's why the Policy of Joint Agreement leads to passionate and frequent sex.

116

GOD CREATED SEX AND MARRIAGE

God not only created marriage, He has also given us the owner's manual, the Bible, in order to know to make it work. And beyond that, He also desires to personally reside in each marriage. God's written Word and personal presence guarantee that any marriage can recover the ecstasy of those early years, even in the midst of the agony.

But first, each married couple must embrace two fundamental realities in God's blueprint for marriage. The seventh biblical purpose for sex is comfort. In 2 Samuel 12:24, David is found comforting his wife when she was grieving. How did he "comfort" her?

By having sex with her. Sometimes in a marriage relationship, it is important for one spouse to generously comfort the other in this way. It shows a genuine love, care, and concern that we can only do for each other.

We need to be grateful as married couples to God for the gift He has given to us to please each other regularly.

Sex is about intimacy, about oneness

When I do this God's way, it is worship. When I do it His way, it is about intimacy (intimacy with my spouse and reflecting intimacy with Him).

When I have sex God's way, it is simply beautiful!

If you are reading this and you are single, would you wait for the one God has for you to be intimate with? If He calls you to singleness, will you let intimacy with Him be enough? If you are single and have already participated in sex outside of God's plan, will you repent and experience God's forgiveness?

If this is you, here are some passages to read:

- Ephesians 2:1-10, and Romans 10:9-10

If you do know Christ:

- 1 John 1:9, and Psalm 51

If you are reading this and are married, would you commit to let sex be about intimacy and about worship of God? If we would do this, then it's very hard to be selfish sexually.

Will we commit to do sex God's way? Will we pursue true sexual intimacy with our spouse if married? Ultimately, will all of us choose to dine with Jesus and have deep intimacy with Him? To do life and sex like this would be an act of worship to God. Are you seeing how these purposes go together?

"A life without love is a waste. 'Should I look for spiritual love, or material, or physical love?', don't ask yourself this question. Discrimination leads to discrimination. Love doesn't need any name, category or definition. Love is a world itself. Either you are in, at the center... either you are out, yearning."

BOTTOM LINE

SEX IS IMPORTANT IN A RELATIONSHIP

It's clear to see that sex is a vital part of any romantic relationship, as well as the relationship's well-being. There are physical benefits, emotional benefits and mental benefits. While we certainly can survive with a lack of sex, most of us won't be thriving.

"Couples often differ in their levels of sexual desire and preferences regarding the frequency of sex, which is something to communicate about, and if there is a major discrepancy (i.e., one partner wants it daily while the other wants it weekly), then a couple must find a happy medium."

"It's also important to note that a healthy sexual relationship centers on communication, consent, and respect, so whatever a couple does sexually, and how often they have sexual interactions, matters less than how they approach their sex life."

To prevent a sexless relationship, it's important that each partner is able to verbalize their needs. "Although the conversation can be hard and awkward, it's necessary." "Lean on the love and care within your relationship to get you through tough conversations." If you need support, it is recommends seeking the help of a sex therapist to guide you.

When God initiates a marital covenant relationship, marriage takes on a sense of the sacred, something uniquely set apart to Him.

By God's design, marriage becomes a binding, contractual relationship, into which He commits Himself to a nurturing role. Husbands and wives are not left alone to hack out their marriage.

No, marriage is a triangle with the husband and wife bound together at the base of the triangle as well as to God who is at the apex of the triangle.

Drawing near to Him will draw them closer to each other.

In other words, marriage is not merely the two becoming one, it is actually the three becoming one: a covenant arrangement of God, the husband, and the wife.

GROW SPIRITUALLY
Knowing that God, through the ministry of the Holy Spirit, is not only a part of your marriage but wants it to succeed for the long haul is encouraging. Also important is understanding that the marital relationship is designed to help us grow spiritually.

The busyness of life can distract us from each other but our individual selfishness can drive us apart.

In a certain sense, every relationship is a transformative relationship, for better or for worse.

"He who walks with wise men will be wise, but the companion of fools will suffer harm" (Prov. 13:20).

"Do not be deceived: 'Bad company corrupts good morals'" (1 Cor. 15:33).

God has committed Himself to changing us into nothing less than the likeness of His Own Son (Rom. 8:29-30; 2 Cor. 3:18).

And that likeness is the likeness of a servant (Phil. 2:5-11).

Marriage is God's ultimate training ground for Christ like servanthood. Most couples are not prepared for the shocking experience of meeting such selfishness in the early months and years of their marriage. Assuming that such selfishness is in their mate, and not in themselves.

They set out with a vengeance to change their mate, usually to no avail. That's when the agony sets in.

But we can only recapture the ecstasy when we begin to realize that we need to be changed, not our mates.

You see, God uses marriage to work out our selfishness and to work in His servanthood.

This is often a slow and painful process.

But God is faithful "who is able to do exceeding abundantly beyond all that we ask or think, according to the power that works within us" (Eph. 3:20).

Moving from agony to ecstasy

Your sexual union faded from ecstasy to agony is not unusual. As one of the most intimate and unifying features of a Christian marriage, our sex life is often symptomatic of our spiritual life.

When we are one with each other and God, we are as close as we can be and sexual excitement is natural expression of this. As we grow spiritually mature together factors like problems at work, family issues and the generally busyness of life are easier to overcome and less likely to take a disproportionate amount of our attention and emotions.

Are you experiences ecstasy or agony in your sex life?

Do you want to transform your marital agony into marital ecstasy? Then take the following steps:

- Reaffirm your marital covenant relationship by committing your marriage to God and to each other in prayer and before another couple who are also living in a committed marital covenant relationship.
- Confess to God that you have been trying to change your mate and that it has been a miserable failure. Also ask your mate to forgive you for trying to play God in your marriage. Ask the Lord to transform you into a Christ like servant in your marriage, no matter what it takes
- Make time to spend together in physical intimacy. Life can get busy, and we can get distracted. Plan times to block out all distractions and just focus one each other.
- Finally, share your prayer requests with another couple who will not only pray for you, but who will also encourage and hold you accountable to these new commitments.